WHAT YOU MUST KNOW ABOUT
THYROID DISORDERS
AND WHAT TO DO ABOUT THEM

PAMELA WARTIAN SMITH, MD, MPH

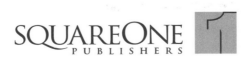

SQUAREONE
PUBLISHERS

EDITORS: Erica Shur and Joanne Abrams
COVER DESIGNER: Jeannie Tudor
TYPESETTER: Gary A. Rosenberg

Square One Publishers
115 Herricks Road
Garden City Park, NY 11040
(516) 535-2010 • (877) 900-BOOK
www.squareonepublishers.com

Library of Congress Cataloging-in-Publication Data
Smith, Pamela Wartian.
  What you must know about thyroid disorders & what to do about them / Dr. Pamela Wartian Smith.
    pages cm
  Includes bibliographical references and index.
  ISBN 978-0-7570-0424-7 (paper) / ISBN 978-0-7570-5424-2 (ebook)
    1. Thyroid gland—Diseases—Popular works. I. Title. II. Title: What you must know about thyroid disorders and what to do about them.
  RC655.S69 2016
  616.4′4—dc23

                                                        2015036248

Printed in the United States of America

10   9   8   7   6   5   4   3

Contents

To my mother,
Bera Avon Hamilton Wartian.
Her passing has helped me understand
that your mother is your connection to the earth.

Acknowledgments

There are many individuals who contributed to this book, particularly my patients who have been my best teachers. Their struggles in battling disease have touched my heart on many occasions.

A special thank you goes to my publisher Rudy Shur. He has been especially important in making this project real. His calming influence, professional direction, and commitment have helped to make the reading of this book flow smoothly. Erica Shur, my editor was instrumental in her editorial contributions. Many thanks, Erica.

Additional and significant thanks goes to my husband, Christopher Smith, who has given me tremendous support in the writing of this book.

Introduction

All the hormones in the body are a symphony. Much like an orchestra, required to play in tune, our hormonal symphony must be in tune throughout your life in order for you to have optimal health. Your thyroid gland is more important than you might think. You are aware that we have a thyroid gland, but chances are that you are not aware of the major role it plays in the complex workings of your body. The thyroid gland regulates most everything that occurs in your system. It is, in fact, the conductor of the wonderful symphony that occurs daily in your body. Commonly, it is not until you experience a thyroid dysfunction that you become aware of how much your thyroid affects your well-being.

The fact that you are reading this book indicates that you may suspect that you or a loved one has a thyroid problem or that a specific thyroid issue has already been identified. If that is the case, I think you've come to the right place. My goal in writing this book is to provide you with an overall understanding of the function of the thyroid gland, the important role the thyroid hormones play in keeping your body functions in tune, and the influence the thyroid gland has on your other body systems. Just as important, it will also offer a closer look at the various problems that arise when the thyroid malfunctions.

The book is divided into ten chapters. Chapter 1 looks at the role the thyroid gland plays as part of the endocrine system—that is, the group of organs and glands responsible for the production of your body's hormones. The text then focuses on the many functions carried on by thyroid hormones and what may occur if they are not at optimal levels. Furthermore, just as important is information on how to maintain a healthy thyroid.

In the following four chapters we examine the specific thyroid disorders. Chapter 2 discusses hypothyroidism, the condition that occurs

1

when the thyroid is underperforming. In Chapter 3, hyperthyroidism, a condition created when the thyroid produces elevated levels of thyroid hormones, is explored. In Chapter 4, Graves' disease, the most common form of hyperthyroidism, is explored. Likewise, in Chapter 5, provided is information on the lesser known forms of hyperthyroidism as well as the various disorders caused by or associated with hyperthyroidism. Within each of these chapters you will learn about their risk factors, their causes, and their signs and symptoms. You will see how a diagnosis for each is derived, and the treatments used for these thyroid disorders. Whenever possible, a prognosis will be provided, in other words, what the likely outcome will be.

The next four chapters will deal with the most common and serious health disorders created as a result of a thyroid problem. Chapter 6 covers thyroid hormones and your memory; Chapter 7, thyroid hormones and your mood; Chapter 8, thyroid hormones and your heart; and Chapter 9, thyroid hormones and digestive health. As you will discover, the role played by thyroid hormones interacting with the heart, brain, and digestive system is critical to your well being.

In Chapter 10, thyroid cancer will be discussed by first explaining what thyroid cancer is. Its risk factors and symptoms will also be elucidated. Because I have found patients can be overwhelmed by not only the situation, but the medical jargon thrown at them, I will explain the terms commonly used to describe the test, characteristics of the cells, the stages, and the treatments provided. I will then discuss each of the most common thyroid cancers. For each I will include risk factors, causes, and signs and symptoms. In addition, I will describe how each is diagnosed, its standard treatments, and its prognosis.

By the end of this book, as you will come to see, although relatively small, the thyroid gland plays a vital role in the human body. Through its release of hormones, it helps regulate heart rate, breathing, digestion, body temperature, weight, mood, memory, and so much more. It is my hope that the information in this book will provide you with all the important facts you may be looking for.

1

You and Your Thyroid

How important is your thyroid gland to your overall health, and what could go wrong with your thyroid gland? What hormones does your thyroid gland produce, and why are they so important? This chapter will address these questions and help you understand how your thyroid gland regulates almost all functions that occur in your body through the production of several hormones. You'll learn how it is instrumental in regulating the body's metabolism and calcium usage; how it affects your brain development, muscle control, heart and digestive function, as well as bone maintenance. The thyroid gland can become overactive (hyperthyroidism) or underactive (hypothyroidism) which affects your well-being resulting in a number of issues, such as weight gain, fatigue, intolerance of hot or cold temperatures, and depression.

You will discover how this butterfly-shaped gland regulates most everything that occurs in your body. A healthy thyroid is essential in order for you to have optimal health. By understanding how the thyroid functions and the various components of the thyroid gland, you will gain insight into the problems created when the thyroid isn't working optimally.

THE ENDOCRINE SYSTEM

The endocrine system is composed of glands and organs (see Figure 1.1) which produce important chemical agents called hormones. This includes the adrenal glands, ovaries, pancreas, parathyroid, pineal gland, pituitary gland, hypothalamus, ovaries and testes, thymus, and thyroid gland, as well as the stomach, small intestines, liver, kidneys, and skin. The hormones produced by the endocrine system regulate the activities of cells and organs in order to help your body function properly. This is done by releasing the hormones directly into the blood stream. When any of these

3

gland's or organ's ability to produce hormones fail to work properly, this can lead to thyroid disease, diabetes, growth disorders, sexual dysfunction, and other serious health issues.

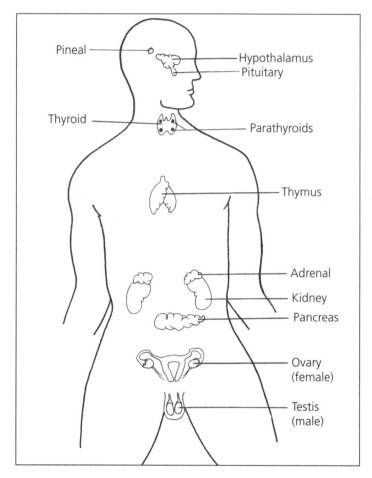

Figure 1.1. The Endocrine System

The hormones released into the blood stream by the glands of the endocrine system are specific to each gland. Each gland performs by releasing hormones that aid in coordinating the body processes.

- Adrenal glands release cortisol and DHEA

- Hypothalamus prompts the pituitary gland to release hormones

- Ovaries release eggs and produce sex hormones

- Pancreas releases the hormones insulin and glucagon

- Parathyroid is crucial to bone development and releases parathyroid hormone

- Pineal gland is linked to patterns of sleep

- Pituitary gland influences many glands, most importantly the thyroid, ovaries, and testes

- Testes produce sperm and sex hormones

- Thymus helps in the development of the immune system early on

- Thyroid controls many aspects of your metabolism, as you will learn

FUNCTIONS OF THE THYROID GLAND AND THYROID HORMONES IN YOUR BODY

The thyroid gland is a key gland producing hormones that play a major part in the human body's everyday workings. These hormones:

- Affect tissue repair and development

- Aid in the function of the mitochondria (energy makers of your cells)

- Assist in the digestion process

- Control hormone secretion

- Control oxygen utilization

- Modulate blood flow

- Regulate carbohydrate, protein, and lipid metabolism

- Modulate muscle and nerve action

- Modulate sexual function

- Regulate energy and heat production

- Regulate growth and repair

- Regulate vitamin usage

Description

Your thyroid gland is one of the largest endocrine glands. It is a ductless gland, butterfly in shape, consisting of two connected lobes (two wings), attached by the isthmus, located in the front of the neck below your Adam's apple, and it is wrapped around the trachea (the windpipe). It is the biggest gland in your neck. It has a brownish-red color as a result of the rich blood vessels located in the thyroid gland. When normal in size,

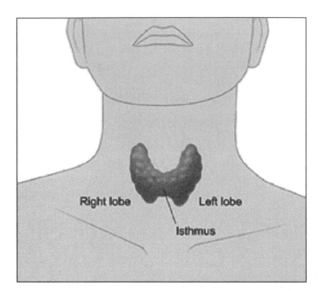

Figure 1.2.
The Thyroid Gland.
Source: National Cancer Institute

you can't feel it. The thyroid is what sets the speed at which your body operates. It reminds your cells to function at a certain rate.

The Thyroid Cells

A healthy thyroid is composed of a number of specialized cells. Many of these cells produce a number of hormones which perform different tasks. Each thyroid cell capable of producing a specific hormone has within it different structures that can identify what type of cell it is, as seen in Table 1.1.

TABLE 1.1 THE NORMAL THYROID CELLS AND THEIR FUNCTION	
Thyroid Cells	**Function**
Follicular cells (epithelial or principal cells)	Cells in the thyroid gland that have control over the production and discharge of thyroid hormones thyroxine (T4) and triiodothyronine (T3). These cells are found lining the surface of the thyroid.
Parafollicular cells (C cells)	Cells that secrete calcitonin (a hormone that regulates calcium metabolism), located in the spaces between the spherical follicles. These cells are large, located in the connective tissue of the thyroid.
Endothelial cells	Cells that are found in the lining of the blood vessels that run through the thyroid.

Hormones and Their Functions

Hormones are chemical agents manufactured by the body. They are produced by specific glands and are secreted into the blood, and then transported by the circulatory system to the areas of the body where they impact cells and organs. Having normal thyroid function relies heavily on the thyroid hormones T2 (3,5-Diiodo-L-thyronine), T3 (Triiodothyronine), T4 (Thyroxin), and rT3 (reverse triiodothyronine) secreted by the thyroid gland. The pituitary gland, located in the brain, is instrumental in the production of these hormones by providing a signal in the form of thyroid stimulating hormone (TSH).

The process begins when the hypothalamus gland, located in the brain, produces the hormone thyrotrophin-releasing hormone (TRH). This in turn stimulates the pituitary gland, also located in the brain, to produce TSH. From the pituitary gland, the TSH travels to the thyroid in order to regulate the production and control the release of each of the thyroid hormones that the body produces. There are several different thyroid hormones that your body synthesizes. They are:

- Diiodothyronine (T2)
- Thyroxine (T4)

- Triiodothyronine (T3)
- Reverse triiodothyronine (rT3)

T2. T2 increases the metabolic rate of your muscles and fat tissues. T2 stimulates cellular/mitochondrial respiration and outside the cell affects the carriers, ion-exchanges, and enzymes. It may also affect the transcription of genes.

T3. This hormone is four to five times more active than T4. T3 is about 20 percent of the thyroid hormone production by the body. It affects most of the physiological processes in the body except for the spleen and testis. This hormone increases basal metabolic rate, oxygen, and energy consumption by the body. It is very important for weight loss and to breakdown cholesterol. It even affects the production of serotonin in the brain which is your happy neurotransmitter. T3 furthermore increases the rate of protein synthesis and affects glucose metabolism.

T4. T4 is 80 percent of the thyroid gland's production. Most of T4 is converted into T3 in your liver or kidneys, so some authors suggest that T4 is really a prohormone (a steroid). T4 is responsible for increasing cardiac output, increasing basal metabolic rate, and increasing heart rate and ventilation. It also potentiates the effect of catecholamines (type of hormone

Conversion of T4 to T3

The hormones T3 and T4 are produced by the follicular cells. The hormone T4 is in "storage" in your body and in order for your body to use T4 it must first change it to the active hormone T3. Deficiencies of zinc, copper, vitamins A, B2, B3, B6, and C are factors that cause decreased production of T4 which leads to symptoms of hypothyroidism. Furthermore, in order for thyroid function to be optimal, your body must easily convert T4 to the more active T3. The conversion of T4 to T3 requires the enzyme 5'deiodinase which plays a role in the activation or deactivation of thyroid hormones. There are three types of 5'deiodinases enzymes which can deiodinate (removal of iodine) thyroid hormones.

- Type I (D1) which is located in the thyroid, liver, and kidney is involved in the production of T3 by converting inactive T4 to active T3

- Type II (D2) which is found in the pituitary, hypothalamus, and brown fat converts T4 to T3

- Type III (D3) which catalyzes deiodination of the inner ring of T4 to T3 inactivates the hormone

As mentioned above deiodinase enzymes are important in the activation or deactivation of thyroid hormones. The following elements affect the production of 5'deiodinase:

- Cadmium, mercury, and lead toxicity
- Chronic illness
- Decreased kidney or liver function
- Elevated cortisol
- High carbohydrate diet
- Inadequate protein intake
- Inflammation
- Selenium deficiency
- Starvation
- Stress

There are numerous factors that affect the conversion of T4 to the more active T3. Although many physicians may prescribe T4 to manage the condition, often this isn't enough. In order to correct the conversion problem, you need to determine what is causing the issue. The following are some common factors that can impede the conversion of T4 to T3.

Nutritional deficiencies

Certain minerals and nutrients are needed to activate enzymes, such as iron, iodine, selenium, zinc, vitamins A, B2, B6, and B12.

Medications

Some medications can interfere with the conversion of T4 to T3. For example:

- Beta blockers
- Clomipramine
- Estrogen replacement
- Glucocorticoids
- Interleukin (IL-6)

- Lithium
- Oral contraceptives
- Some chemotherapeutic agents
- Theophylline

Diet

Your diet may be a crucial element in the conversion process as well and can negatively impact thyroid production.

- Eating too many walnuts
- Excessive alcohol use
- Low carbohydrate diet
- Low fat diet

- Low protein diet
- Large amount of soy
- Too many cruciferous vegetables (broccoli, cauliflower, kale, Brussels sprouts)

Other factors that inhibit the T4 to T3 conversion

- Aging process
- Calcium excess
- Copper excess
- Diabetes
- Dioxins
- Fluoride
- High dose alpha lipoic acid (600 mg and above)
- Inadequate production DHEA and/or cortisol

- Lead
- Mercury
- PCBs
- Pesticides
- Phthalates (chemicals added to plastics)
- Radiation
- Stress
- Surgery

that strongly affects blood pressure) and thickens the endometrium of the uterus in women. T4 can also be converted into rT3 which is an inactive (stored) form.

rT3. Reverse T3 is produced from T4 and its function is to block the action of T3. Chronic stress (as well as the factors that follow) causes the adrenal glands to manufacture a high level of cortisol which hinders the conversion of T4 to T3 and may result in an increased rT3. This is a measurement of inactive thyroid function. Your rT3 has only one percent of the activity T3 does. It is an antagonist of T3, which means that the higher your rT3 level is the lower your T3 level will be. T3 and rT3 bind to the same receptor sites, so they cannot both occupy these sites at the same time. This situation occurs due to a malfunction of the metabolism of T4. The following are factors that are associated with low T3 or increased reverse T3:

- Aging process
- Diabetes
- Elevated levels of IL-6, TNF-alpha, IFN-2
- Fasting
- Free radical production
- Increased levels of epinephrine and/or norepinephrine
- Prolonged illness
- Stress
- Toxic metal exposure

When rT3 is high this is a medical syndrome now called "rT3 dominance."

Causes of rT3 Dominance

The rT3 dominance, also known as Wilson's Syndrome, is a condition exhibiting hypothyroid symptoms. The causes of this condition include:

- Autoimmune disease
- Exposure to electromagnetic radiation
- Exposure to environmental toxins, such as chemical pollutants, pesticides, mercury, or fluoride
- Food deprivation
- High levels of stress
- Hormonal imbalance (such as high estrogen levels in women)
- Infections
- Nutritional deficiencies
- Poor liver function

Furthermore, high normal or elevated rT3 is indicative of reduced thyroid transport. It may cause your metabolism to slow down, affecting your body temperature, fatigue, and eating habits. This is due to mitochondrial dysfunction. Your body needs energy to carry out its many jobs. If you suffer from mitochondrial dysfunction the mitochondria in the cells are not changing nutrients into energy, and therefore needed energy is not produced. Hence, any disease process associated with mitochondrial dysfunction may be associated with high normal or elevated rT3. There are several conditions that have been found to be commonly associated with elevated rT3.

- Aging
- Anxiety
- Bipolar depression
- Cardiovascular disease
- Chronic and acute dieting
- Chronic fatigue syndrome
- Chronic infections
- Depression
- Diabetes
- Fibromyalgia
- Hypercholesterolemia (high cholesterol) and hypertriglyceridemia (high triglycerides)
- Inflammation and chronic illnesses
- Insulin resistance
- Migraines
- Neurodegenerative disorders such as Parkinson's disease and Alzheimer's disease
- Obesity

When you have a high rT3 level, you may have symptoms of low thyroid function (hypothyroidism). When your rT3 level is high your body temperature goes down. This slows the action of many enzymes in your body which can lead to a syndrome called "multiple enzyme dysfunction."

Symptoms of Multiple Enzyme Dysfunction

- Anxiety
- Fatigue
- Fluid retention
- Headache
- Irritability
- Migraine headaches
- Panic attacks
- PMS

The transporter for T4 is more energy dependent than the transporter for T3. Cellular levels of thyroid are not detected well by serum T4 levels since serum T4 is transported into the cell and the lower the cellular level of T4 the higher the serum level. The most important determinant of thyroid activity is the intra-cellular T3 level. High normal or elevated rT3 levels are the best measure of thyroid transport into the cell. Furthermore, consider looking at free T3 to rT3 ratio.

Lab Studies to Evaluate Thyroid Function

Conditions that interfere with the normal process of the thyroid gland are categorized as influencing the thyroid directly or indirectly. Blood tests

TABLE 1.2 THYROID FUNCTION TEST INTERPRETATION		
Test	Normal Range*	Possible Diagnosis
TSH	0.3 to 2.0	High TSH indicates an underactive thyroid (hypothyroidism)
		Low TSH indicates an overactive thryroid (hyperthyroidism)
Free T4	0.7 to 2	Levels are low (hypothyroidism)
		Levels are elevated (hyperthyroidism)
Free T3	2.3 to 4.2	Levels are elevated (hyperthyroidism)
		Levels are low (hypothyroidism)
rT3		Levels elevated (triggered by chronic stress, pneumonia, injury, surgery, low-iron, or low-cortisol) (hypothyroidism or hyperthyroidism)
Thyroid antibodies:		Normal range should be negative
Antithyroglobulin	Negative	Positive indicates Hashimoto's thyroiditis
Antimicrosomal	Negative	Positive indicates Hashimoto's thyroiditis, autoimmune hemolytic anemia, Graves' disease, Sjogren syndrome, systemic lupus erythematosus, rheumatoid arthritis, and/or thyroid cancer
Antithyroperoxidase (ATPO)	Negative	Positive indicates Hashimoto's thyroiditis, Graves' disease, Sjogren's syndrome, lupus, rheumatoid arthritis, and/or pernicious anemia

*Normal range may vary from lab to lab.

are readily available and widely used to measure thyroid function and identify the most common causes of thyroid dysfunction. Blood analyses are used to determine whether or not your thyroid is functioning properly. It is very important that you have optimal levels of thyroid hormone and not just normal levels. See Table 1.2 on page 12 for a list of your normal thyroid hormones based on your blood test, as well as the optimal range of thyroid hormone for each lab.

Standard Blood Test. Normally, every blood test you take includes a group of tests that look at your body's hormones. It typically analyzes your thyroid hormones including TSH, T3, T4, and the thyroid hormones Antithyroglobulin, Antimicrosomal, and Antithyroperoxidase. The results are printed on your blood test lab report.

Thyroid Binding Globulin Test (TBG). This test is specifically administered to find the reason for elevated or diminished levels of thyroid hormone. The thyroid binding globulin:

- Stores thyroid hormone

- Is produced in the liver

- Is affected by illness, liver disease, and medications

- Estrogen replacement can increase TBG proteins

Thyrotropin-releasing Hormone Test (TRH). This test is specifically to find the levels of the thyrotropin-releasing hormone, also called thyrotropin-releasing factor (TRF):

- Stimulates the release of TSH and prolactin from the pituitary

- Is produced by hypothalamus

- Is the central regulator of the hypothalamic-pituitary-thyroid (HPT) axis

- Has affects independent of the HPT axis

- As you age the body commonly produces less TRH which is implicated in neurodegenerative diseases (Alzheimer's and Parkinson's)

- Protects the neurons against oxidative stress, glutamate toxicity, caspase-induced cell death, DNA fragmentation, and inflammation

- Involved in immune regulation

MAINTAINING A HEALTHY THYROID GLAND

Although many thyroid disorders may be genetic, you can greatly *reduce* the risk of developing any thyroid malfunctions by paying close attention to the foods you eat, making sure you get enough exercise, and avoiding as many toxins as you can.

Diet

A diet that is balanced and rich in vitamin A, iodine, selenium, and iron will aid in hormone production. To increase your selenium intake choose foods, such as Brazil nuts, shellfish, mushrooms, wheat germ, sunflower and sesame seeds, onion, garlic, beef liver, and eggs. The daily recommended dose is as follows:

- Vitamin A: 4,000 IU daily

- Iodine: People age 14 and older, 150 mcg daily

- Iron: For men 8 mg daily, for women 18 mg up to menopause, after menopause take 8 mg daily

- Selenium: Daily dose 55 mcg, however try to get the daily requirement from the foods listed above

Considerations

- Sugar intake interferes with a balanced diet, since sugar provides "empty calories." Sugar can reduce thyroid function, lower circulation, and also cause weight gain.

- Polyunsaturated oils should be limited as well, as they affect hormone and progesterone production. Replacing polyunsaturated oils with coconut oil is a healthy choice.

- Monitor foods that suppress the function of the thyroid gland by interfering with the absorption of iodine, for example green cruciferous vegetables (broccoli, Brussel sprouts, collard greens, spinach, kale, and others), as well as certain fruits, such as peaches, pears, and strawberries. These foods should be eaten in moderation unless you already have a low iodine level.

Exercise

Physical activity is instrumental in achieving a healthy body weight, it will decrease stress levels, increase lean muscle mass, and provide you with more energy. Aerobic exercise can raise your levels of T3 and T4, for those who suffer from low levels of thyroid hormones, and boost your metabolism. A regular exercise program and staying active is important for circulation which is essential in assisting the thyroid in the distribution of hormones.

Limiting Exposure to Synthetic Hormones

Many people do not realize that they come into contact with synthetic hormones and hormone-like chemicals in daily living. For example, synthetic estrogen may be derived from animal estrogen. The body recognizes these type of hormones as foreign substances and does not metabolize them well. Unfortunately, there are a number of synthetic hormones in the things that you come into contact with every day that may have a detrimental effect on your thyroid health. Xenoestrogens are a type of synthetic hormone that imitates estrogen and has been implicated in many conditions. They pass into the environment and into your body through certain foods, plastics, certain chemicals, and household and personal products.

Synthetic hormones may increase your risk of developing heart disease, breast cancer, ovarian cancer, high blood pressure, and so on. You cannot totally avoid xenoestrogens, but you can lessen their effect and the chances of being exposed to them.

Considerations

- Drinking filtered water rather than tap water
- Eating organic foods that have not been exposed to pesticides and herbicides rather than processed foods that may contain preservatives and synthetic hormones
- Using natural detergents and body care products
- Decreasing caffeine intake may improve your thyroid function
- Using organic household cleaning products

Annual Medical Check-Ups

Diet, exercise, and limiting exposure to synthetic hormones can help you maintain a healthy thyroid and alleviate the symptoms of some thyroid conditions, but it should not be a substitute for a medical examination and blood test. By learning what the signs and symptoms of the most common thyroid problems are, you will be in a better position to have them evaluated by your physician and catch it early enough to stop it from causing serious harm to your body. In Table 1.3 you will find the most common thyroid disorders that are often related to an over- or an under-functioning thyroid.

TABLE 1.3 DISORDERS AND THEIR RELATED HORMONE ISSUES	
Disorder	**Hormone Issue**
Goiter	Iodine deficiency, excess production of thyroid hormone
Hashimoto's Thyroiditis	Low production of thyroid hormone
Hyperthyroidism	High production of thyroid hormone
Hypothyroidism	Low production of thyroid hormone
Graves' Disease	Excess production of thyroid hormone
Thyroid Cancer	Iodine deficiency, low level of thyroid hormone promotes higher production of TSH which promotes growth of thyroid cancer cells (See Chapter 8.)
Thyroid Nodule	Excess of thyroid hormone, diets deficient in iodine
Thyroid Storm (a medical emergency condition)	Excess of thyroid hormone, over-replacement of thyroid hormone

CONCLUSION

As you can see, your thyroid gland is one of the most important glands in your body since it is the conductor of your body's symphony. In order for you to have optimal health, your thyroid gland, along with your hypothalamus and pituitary gland which help regulate thyroid hormone production, must all be functioning perfectly. In the next chapter you will learn about the causes, symptoms, and the treatment of a low functioning thyroid gland, a condition referred to as hypothyroidism.

2

Hypothyroidism and Hashimoto's Thyroiditis

ypothyroidism—an underactive thyroid—is a more common disorder than you may think. As of 2014 the American Association of Clinical Endocrinologists (AACCE) has cited that about 27 million Americans suffer from thyroid disease. Of these, around 80 percent of them are women. People of any age can suffer from hypothyroidism, but it is more common in older adults. The AACCE has stated that a woman is 5 to 8 times more inclined to have an underactive thyroid than a man, and women over the age of 50 are at a higher risk. While hypothyroidism can take several forms, the most common is Hashimoto's thyroiditis. (See page 36 for details.)

HYPOTHYROIDISM

Hypothyroidism is defined as low thyroid function or an underactive thyroid where the thyroid gland does not make enough thyroid hormones to allow the body to function optimally. The main function of the thyroid hormone is to oversee your metabolism, therefore people with this condition have symptoms associated with a low functioning metabolism. Hypothyroidism disturbs the normal equilibrium of the chemical reactions in the body. Unfortunately, the earliest signs and symptoms of low thyroid function can occur several years prior to laboratory results being abnormal. It is therefore important to be aware of this disorder's signs and symptoms.

RISK FACTORS

There are a number of risk factors that can increase the possibility of developing hypothyroidism. The following elements may indicate if an individual is at increased risk:

Age

Although hypothyroidism can occur at any age, women over the age of 60 are more likely to develop hypothyroidism.

Autoimmune Disorders

Medical research has found that 90 percent of people produce antibodies that attack and destroy thyroid tissue. This process over time limits the amount of thyroid hormones being produced, which leads to hypothyroidism.

Genetics

Statistics strongly indicate that genetics plays a role in a person's predisposition to developing hypothyroidism. While there is no evidence that only one gene is to blame, it is more likely that the presence of several specific genes increase the incidence of hypothyroidism. However in order to turn these genes on, it may require one or more triggers, as listed below, to initiate this condition.

Gender

Women are at a higher risk of developing hypothyroidism then men.

Ethnicity

Statistically, whites or Asians appear to be at greater risk for hypothyroidism than other people.

CAUSES OF HYPOTHYROIDISM

The cause of hypothyroidism is commonly due to a problem with the thyroid gland. Less common etiologies may be related to problems in the hypothalamus or the pituitary gland. In addition, hypothyroidism may be due to a number of other factors, such as diet, Hashimoto's thyroiditis (see page 36), an unhealthy gut, thyroid surgery, radiation therapy, and medications, as well as deficiencies in certain minerals and vitamins, which are factors that cause decreased production of T4 and lead to symptoms of hypothyroidism.

Diet

Some studies suggest that a diet high in soy may actually decrease thyroid function. Natural-occurring chemicals in soy may interfere with the absorption of thyroid hormones that you may be taking. This is controversial in the medical literature, but if you are on a high soy diet, and you are suffering from a thyroid problem, then you may want to decrease or stop your soy intake to see if it improves your thyroid function.

Naturally occurring chemicals are contained in some vegetables that may disrupt normal function of the thyroid. Additionally, foods grown in nutritionally depleted soil may be deficient in important vitamins and minerals. (See related sections on nutritional deficiencies that follow.)

Iodine Deficiency

Iodine deficiency is a major cause of hypothyroidism. Iodine has therapeutic actions in the body. It is an antibacterial, anticancer, antiparasitic, antiviral, and mucolytic agent. The thyroid gland uses iodine on a daily basis. Iodine deficiency may affect other organs in the body as well, such as kidneys, breasts, prostate, spleen, liver, blood, salivary glands, and intestines.

There are many causes of iodine deficiency including the following:

- Food grown in iodine-depleted soil

- Diets without ocean fish or sea vegetables such as seaweed

- Inadequate use of iodized salt (low salt diet) in a region such as the Midwest which is low in iodine

- Diet that is high in pasta and breads which contain bromide (bromide binds to iodine receptors and prevents iodine from binding)

- Fluoride use (inhibits iodine binding)

- Vegan and vegetarian diets

- Sucralose (artificial sweetener that contains chlorinated table sugar)

- Medications (the following are some examples, but any medication that contains bromide or fluoride can lead to iodine deficiency)

  - Atrovent inhaler (contains bromide)

  - Ipratropium nasal spray (contains bromide)

  - Pro-panthine (contains bromide)

- Flonase (contains fluoride)
- Flovent (contains fluoride)

If you are on one of these medications do not discontinue their use. Instead see your health care provider and have your iodine levels measured to see if you are deficient in iodine. Then your physician can make appropriate recommendations.

The Importance of Iodine

Iodine is essential for everyone. It is a chemical element that is crucial for good health. Many conditions beside hypothyroidism may be improved with iodine supplementation including:

- Dupuytren's contracture
- Excess mucous production
- Fatigue

- Fibrocystic breast disease
- Headaches/migraine headaches
- Hemorrhoids

- Keloids
- Ovarian cysts
- Parotid duct stones
- Peyronie's disease
- Sebaceous cysts

Breast health is related to iodine levels. Studies have shown that areas of the world with high iodine intake like Japan have a lower rate of breast cancer.

According to the World Health Organization, up to 72 percent of the world's population is affected by an iodine deficiency disorder. If you are allergic to shell fish, then you are probably are allergic to iodine and should not supplement with it. If you take thyroid hormone and you then start taking iodine you may need less thyroid medication, therefore it is best if you have your iodine levels measured before you start on thyroid hormone. In fact, sometimes your symptoms of hypothyroidism may resolve and your labs may normalize with just taking iodine if you are low in this important nutrient. Most people do better when they take iodine supplements to take both iodine and iodide as one preparation. Lugol's solution would be one way of doing this. It is a liquid but has a metallic taste so you may opt to take the iodine/iodine supplement as a pill.

It is very important that you have your iodine levels measured before you start taking iodine. Too much iodine in the diet, or by supplementation, has been associated with thyroiditis which is an inflammation of your thyroid gland. High levels of iodine can cause it to be trapped by thyroglobulin. Elevated levels of iodinated thyroglobulin then prompt the immune system to react and to cause inflammation. Furthermore, research has shown that in some areas of the world where there is high dietary iodine content or excessive supplementation that there is also an increase in not just thyroiditis but also thyroid cancer. Therefore it is important that you have your iodine levels measured before you begin iodine replacement. If you are on an iodine supplement, taking vitamin B2 (Riboflavin) and vitamin B3 (Niacin) helps make the iodine easier for the thyroid gland to absorb. Some studies suggest that if you have Hashimoto's thyroiditis (see page 36) that you should not supplement with iodine. More research needs to be done on this subject.

Iron Deficiency

One of the issues that may result from of an underactive thyroid is iron deficiency. In order for your thyroid to function optimally you have to have enough iron in your body. When the thyroid is underactive, the red blood cell production drops. It also plays a part in T4 to T3 conversion. In addition, iron is necessary for optimal immune system health, which is important if you are suffering from Graves' disease or Hashimoto's thyroiditis. Iron deficiency can be caused by the following:

- Loss of blood

- Consuming too little iron

- Body's inability to absorb iron

- For women, pregnancy and blood loss during the menstrual cycle

Women are more likely to be deficient in iron, especially in their childbearing years.

Magnesium Deficiency

Magnesium is an important supplement since most people are deficient in this mineral. Seven out of every ten Americans suffer from magnesium deficiency. Although there are several symptoms that may result from magnesium deficiency, the most common one is low thyroid function. Magnesium is necessary for the proper absorption of iodine. In addition, although magnesium is essential to every organ in your body, it is particularly important in the function of the heart, kidneys, and muscles.

Magnesium deficiency can result when you take large doses of vitamin C. The problem being that vitamin C competes with magnesium. In addition, healthy thyroid function relies on a balance of calcium and magnesium in the body.

Other causes of magnesium deficiency include:

- Alcohol abuse
- Certain medications
- Diarrhea
- Eating a diet high in trans fatty acids
- Excessive sugar intake
- Extreme athletic competition
- Gastrointestinal disorders
- High caffeine intake
- Increased consumption of foods and drinks high in oxalic acid (such as almonds, cocoa, spinach, and tea)
- Minimal intake of foods rich in magnesium
- Phosphates in soft drinks
- Poor absorption
- Stress
- Surgery
- Taking magnesium supplements while eating a high fiber meal
- Trauma

Selenium Deficiency

The mineral selenium is very important for your general health, as well as for your thyroid gland and thyroid hormones to function properly in your body. A deficiency in selenium can affect the conversion process of T4 to T3. Selenium deficiency can be rare, however it can develop under certain conditions. The following are some of these circumstances:

- Foods that are grown on poor selenium soils
- Malabsorption, especially in the very elderly
- Severe gastrointestinal disorders

Vitamin B Deficiency

A deficiency in vitamin B2 can contribute to a low functioning thyroid. A lack of vitamin B2 suppresses the production of T4 and keeps the thyroid and adrenal glands from secreting their hormones. Vitamin B3 is needed to keep the endocrine cells in efficient working order. It plays a role in the production of thyroid hormones. Vitamin B3 is needed to produce tyrosine (an amino acid) in the body, and T3 and T4 are derived from tyrosine. Also, be aware that taking vitamin B2 (riboflavin) and vitamin B3 (niacin) is crucial if you are on iodine supplementation. It is also important in maintaining a healthy thyroid.

Vitamin D Deficiency

Like magnesium, many people are not aware that they have low levels of Vitamin D. Low levels of Vitamin D may interfere with the thyroid functioning properly. If you are suffering from an autoimmune thyroid condition, you can benefit from being tested for a deficiency in vitamin D. You can request your Vitamin D level to be checked when you have your next blood test. Besides taking daily vitamin D supplements, daily exposure to the sun is beneficial.

Zinc Deficiency

Without the existence of zinc in the body the thyroid cannot convert the less active hormone T4 to the active hormone T3. The hypothalamus also depends upon zinc to make the hormone it uses to cue the pituitary gland to switch on the thyroid. Too little zinc may lead to a low functioning thyroid. In fact, zinc is a cofactor in over 100 reactions in the body. Chronic zinc deficiency can weaken your immune system.

Medications

Sometimes medications or nutrients are associated with a decrease in thyroid function. They may affect the thyroid function if your thyroid is intact or if you are on thyroid medication. The following agents lower absorption of thyroid hormone or elevate the excretion of thyroid hormone:

- Aluminum hydroxide
- Bile acid sequestrants
- Calcium
- Ferrous sulfate
- Lactose
- Sucralfate

The following are other medications that may also alter thyroid function:

- Amiodarone (inhibit conversion of T4 to T3)
- Cimetidine (can modify peripheral metabolism of thyroid hormones)
- Clomiphene
- Haloperidol
- Lithium (blocks iodine transport)
- Metoclopramide
- Oral contraceptives

There are also medications that increase the clearance of thyroid hormone so that it leaves the body sooner, such as:

- Carbamezapine
- Phenobarbitol
- Phenytoin
- Rifampin
- Ritonavir
- Sertraline
- Tamoxifen used for more than one year

For those who rely on treatment with thyroid hormone medicine, taking certain supplements, for example calcium or iron, at the same time as the thyroid medication may decrease the amount of thyroid medicine that is being absorbed. It is recommended that calcium and iron supplements should not be taken at the same time as the thyroid hormone medication.

SIGNS AND SYMPTOMS OF HYPOTHYROIDISM

Early diagnosis of hypothyroidism isn't always easy. Most people with an underactive thyroid aren't aware that they have this condition. They may suffer a number of symptoms without recognizing that the symptoms are thyroid-related or that there may be no symptoms early on in the disease process. Often times, the physician may minimize or misdiagnose the symptoms. The signs and symptoms of hypothyroidism normally progress slowly, over months or years, and quite often they may be confused with other disorders. The following are signs and symptoms of hypothyroidism:

- ❏ Acne
- ❏ Agitation/irritability
- ❏ Allergies
- ❏ Anxiety/panic attacks
- ❏ Arrhythmias (irregular heart rhythm)
- ❏ Bladder and kidney infections
- ❏ Blepharospasm (eye twitching) is more common
- ❏ Carpal tunnel syndrome
- ❏ Cholesterol levels that are high (hypercholesterolemia)
- ❏ Cognitive decline
- ❏ Cold hands and feet
- ❏ Cold intolerance
- ❏ Congestive heart failure
- ❏ Constipation
- ❏ Coronary heart disease/acute myocardial infarction (heart attack)
- ❏ Decreased cardiac output
- ❏ Decreased sexual interest
- ❏ Delayed deep tendon reflexes
- ❏ Deposition of mucin (glyco-protein) in connective tissues
- ❏ Depression
- ❏ Dizziness/vertigo
- ❏ Downturned mouth
- ❏ Drooping eyelids
- ❏ Dull facial expression
- ❏ Ear canal that is dry, scaly, and may itch
- ❏ Ear wax build-up in the ear canal (cerumen)
- ❏ Easy bruising
- ❏ Eating disorders
- ❏ Elbows that are rough and bumpy (keratosis)
- ❏ Endometriosis
- ❏ Erectile dysfunction
- ❏ "Fat pads" above the clavicles
- ❏ Fatigue
- ❏ Fibrocystic breast disease
- ❏ Fluid retention
- ❏ Gallstones
- ❏ Hair loss in the front and back of the head
- ❏ Hair loss in varying amounts from legs, axilla, and arms
- ❏ Hair that is sparse, coarse, and dry
- ❏ Headaches, including migraine headaches
- ❏ High cortisol levels
- ❏ High C-reactive protein (CRP)
- ❏ Hoarse, husky voice
- ❏ High homocysteine levels (hyperhomocysteinemia)
- ❏ High insulin levels (hyperinsulinemia)
- ❏ Hypertension (high blood pressure)
- ❏ Hypoglycemia (low blood sugar)
- ❏ Impaired kidney function

- ❏ Inability to concentrate
- ❏ Increased appetite
- ❏ Increased risk of developing asthma
- ❏ Increased risk of developing bipolar disorder
- ❏ Increased risk of developing schizoid or affective psychoses
- ❏ Infertility
- ❏ Insomnia
- ❏ Iron deficiency anemia
- ❏ Joint stiffness (arthralgias)
- ❏ Loss of eyelashes or eyelashes that are not as thick
- ❏ Loss of one-third of the eyebrows
- ❏ Low amplitude theta and delta brain waves.
- ❏ Low blood pressure
- ❏ Low body temperature
- ❏ Menstrual cycle pain
- ❏ Menstrual irregularities including abnormally heavy bleeding
- ❏ Mild elevation of liver enzymes
- ❏ Miscarriage
- ❏ Morning stiffness
- ❏ Muscle and joint pain
- ❏ Muscle craps
- ❏ Muscle weakness
- ❏ Muscular pain
- ❏ Nails that are brittle, easily broken, ridged, striated, thickened nails
- ❏ Nocturia (need to get up and urinate in the middle of the night)
- ❏ Nutritional imbalances
- ❏ Osteoporosis (bone loss)
- ❏ Paresthesia (abnormal sensation of feeling burning, tingling, and itching)
- ❏ Poor circulation
- ❏ Poor night vision
- ❏ Premenstrual syndrome (PMS)
- ❏ Puffy face
- ❏ Reduced heart rate
- ❏ Rough, dry skin
- ❏ Shortness of breath
- ❏ Sleep apnea
- ❏ Slow movements
- ❏ Slow speech
- ❏ Swollen eyelids
- ❏ Swollen legs, feet, hands, and abdomen
- ❏ Tendency to develop allergies
- ❏ Tinnitus (ringing in the ears)
- ❏ Vitamin B12 deficiency
- ❏ Weight gain
- ❏ Yellowish skin discoloration due to the inability to convert beta carotene into vitamin A

There are some conditions that may be or may not be signs and symptoms of hypothyroidism, such as growth hormone deficiency in children, retrograde uterus, vitiligo, skin cancer, dry eyes, TMJ, and teeth clenching. If you suffer from any one or a number of these health issues, and no root cause has been found to alleviate the problem, perhaps it's time to consider looking at how well your thyroid is functioning.

DIAGNOSIS

Early detection of hypothyroidism is not always easy. However, there are a number of steps you can take to discover if you are suffering from an underactive thyroid. This process can incorporate several factors, such as clinical evaluation and blood tests. In addition, since a thyroid condition or disease may encompass many factors, other tests may be administered as well, such as imaging tests and biopsies.

Self-Awareness

As you have seen on page 24, there are many signs and symptoms associated with the underproduction of thyroid hormones. A lack of these key chemicals can cause many health issues to occur. If you see that you suffer from a number of these problems, you can conduct a simple home test to see if there is a possibility of you having this condition.

Home Testing

If you are experiencing specific signs or symptoms that indicate you may have an underactive thyroid (see page 24), you can administer a safe and simple home test (see inset on page 28). You can determine the possibility of any potential thyroid dysfunction on your own, at your home, by measuring you basal temperature. Although this test is obviously not an official diagnosis of a thyroid dysfunction, it can give you some indication that you need to follow up with your physician for further testing to be administered.

Consult With Your Doctor

If you feel a problem does exist, it is very important that you see your health care provider for an evaluation of your thyroid gland; and, that you have a complete workup done and not a partial workup.

Simple Home Tests to Determine If You Have a Potential Problem

The thyroid gland can be thought of as the body's thermostat. The hormones produced by the thyroid play a role in keeping you warm. Some patients will have normal or even optimal levels of thyroid hormone, but they still will have symptoms of hypothyroidism. For these individuals it is important to get a basal body temperature, since keeping the body at its optimal temperature setting cannot be achieved when the thyroid is struggling.

By measuring your basal temperature yourself at home, you can determine if you have a thyroid issue. A basal body temperature is the temperature taken underneath your arm.

1. Place a mercury type thermometer within reach before bedtime.

2. Shake it down until you reach 96 degrees Fahrenheit.

3. Before you arise in the morning as soon as you awake place the thermometer under your armpit for 10 minutes.

4. You take your temperature for three consecutive days and record the temperature.

A normal temperature is 97.8 to 98.2 degrees Fahrenheit. If you have an underactive thyroid, your average temperature will be lower than 97.8 degrees Fahrenheit. If you are a menstruating woman, then take your temperature during your menstrual cycle.

Clinical Evaluation

Your physician will perform a complete physical exam of the gland, where he/she palpates your thyroid to determine if there are any lumps, nodules, growths (goiters), or masses. In addition, he/she will be checking the thyroid's size, and if it is solid and firmly fixed in place.

Blood Tests

The blood test is the most common test, and plays an important role in diagnosing thyroid disease and treating thyroid conditions. A number of blood tests will be done in order to determine if you are suffering from hypothyroidism. Your physician will be evaluating your TSH, free T4, freeT3, rt3 (reverse T3), and thyroid antibodies (see Table 1.2 on page 12).

Thyroid binding globulin (TBG) can also be measured (see page 13). This is the amount of stored hormone. It is produced by the liver and is affected by illness, liver disease, and some medications. Sometimes estrogens can raise TBG, so this is another test that your doctor may order. Your health care provider may also order thyroid releasing hormone (TRH) also called thyrotropin-releasing factor (TRF) which is a hormone that stimulates the release of thyroid stimulating hormone (TSH) and prolactin from the pituitary. (See page 13.)

Some people have an autoimmune process where their body is literally trying to attack its own thyroid gland and the body produces a normal amount of thyroid hormone or not enough thyroid hormone. This is called Hashimoto's thyroiditis. Your test results will reveal that your thyroid antibody levels are high. (See Table 1.2 on page 12.)

Imaging Tests

Laboratory tests may not be enough to diagnosis thyroid dysfunction. Sometimes more tests are ordered. Imaging tests are administered for a diagnosis of various thyroid disorders. The following are other tests that may be performed:

- Iodine Uptake Scan: to measure the absorption of iodine in the thyroid.

- Thyroid Scan: a radioisoptope is administered, usually given with the iodine uptake. Cells that do not absorb iodine will appear "cold (lighter on the scan)," a cell absorbing too much iodine will appear "hot (darker)."

- Thyroid Ultrasound: high frequency sound waves provide an image of the thyroid gland. It aids in performing fine need biopsies.

Fine Needle Aspiration (FNA)

Fine needle aspiration is a type of biopsy procedure that is commonly performed to detect or rule out cancer cells in the thyroid. It is commonly performed on swellings or lumps found in the thyroid. The fine needle aspiration can identify the type of cells contained in the abnormal tissue or fluid. (See Chapter 3 on page 49)

TREATMENT OF HYPOTHYROIDISM

There are several things to consider in looking at treatment for low thyroid function. You may benefit from detoxification of the liver or helping your gut stay healthy. You may have nutritional deficiencies and improving your nutritional status may improve your thyroid function. You may be taking a medication that causes your thyroid not to function as well as it could. This does not mean that you should stop your medication, but it does mean that certain medications may cause your thyroid not to function optimally, and you may have to replace a nutrient that is deplete due to a medication or you may have to take thyroid medication due to another drug that you are taking. Lastly, you may benefit from thyroid replacement as a medication.

Detoxification

Sometimes individuals with hypothyroidism do not need medication but would benefit from a quality detoxification program. There is evidence that elements in the environment and diet can lead to thyroid conditions. You can treat these thyroid problems by detoxing your thyroid. PCBs, dioxins, DDT, HCB (hexachlorobenzene), phthalates, and high levels of heavy metals, such as lead, arsenic, and mercury can cause dysfunction of your thyroid gland; affecting both the production and conversion of thyroid hormones. It is possible to measure levels of most of these toxins and then work on their removal. Cleaning out many of the toxins will not only address your thyroid symptoms, but it will give you an overall sense of well-being and good health. If you have never used detoxification supplements it may be wise to consult with a doctor first.

With any detoxification program you need to follow certain guidelines to make it most effective.

- Take a quality cleansing product

- Eat healthy and avoid refined foods, sugars, and junk food

- Drink purified water and avoid alcohol, sodas, and sugar drinks

- Be sure that you are eliminating the toxins

After your first detoxification program it is recommended that you go through detoxification once a year. (See also Diet below.)

The 4R program (Remove, Replace, Reinnoculate, and Repair) is an effective way to stabilize and treat gastrointestinal dysfunction and to further gastrointestinal health (see Chapter 6). Sometimes when the patient's GI tract health is improved by using the 4R program they no longer have symptoms of hypothyroidism and their labs also normalize.

Diet

Besides supplements, your diet and the kinds of foods you consume can provide you with some of the nutrients needed for a healthy thyroid gland. Whether or not you need a nutrient supplement in addition to your diet can be determined by a blood test that will indicate where you are deficient. Fortunately there are supplements, herbs, and nutrients that can boost the conversion of T4 to T3. The following may be considered:

- Ashwaganda (an herb)
- High protein diet
- Iodine
- Iron
- Melatonin
- Potassium
- Replacement of testosterone in men (decreases the concentration of thyroid binding globulin)
- Selenium
- Tyrosine (an amino acid)
- Vitamins A, B2, E
- Zinc

Some studies have shown that a diet high in soy may decrease thyroid function. This is controversial in the medical literature, but if you are on a high soy diet then you may want to decrease your soy intake to see if it improves your thyroid function.

A diet consisting of processed foods and sodas leads to magnesium deficiency. Foods that are rich in magnesium consist of nuts and seeds, legumes, meats, and grains, such as rice and oats.

Iron can be found in foods such as meat, fish, and poultry, and the iron found in these foods is absorbed easily. Plant based foods, such as nuts, vegetables, grains, and fruits are less absorbable. To keep your ferritin (a protein in the body that binds iron) levels at normal range it is crucial to either get enough iron from the foods you eat or from a supplement or from both.

To ensure that you are consuming a rich source of vitamin B2 you should include meat, mushrooms, almonds, whole grains, and leafy green vegetables in your diet. Foods high in vitamin B3 are chicken and turkey, beef, and pine nuts. Some dietary sources of vitamin D include fish liver oils, beef liver, egg, alfalfa, and mushrooms. The mineral zinc can be found in protein rich foods, such as meat, nuts, legumes, seafood, and whole grains.

If you have high or positive thyroid antibodies then the best thing that you can do is to stop ingesting any gluten. The next best thing that you can do is to help your gastrointestinal tract (GI tract) be healthier (see chapter 6.)

Supplementation

There are a number of nutritional supplements you can take to stabilize your thyroid gland and restore its function, such as iodine, magnesium, selenium, vitamin B, vitamin D, and zinc. A deficiency in any of these nutrients can negatively affect your health. Not everyone with a hypothyroidism is deficient in the same nutrients, therefore it is necessary to be tested to diagnose what you may be deficient in. If you are deficient in basic nutrients, then starting a multivitamin may help your thyroid function improve.

Iodine. Iodine has therapeutic actions in the body. It is an antibacterial, anticancer, antiparasitic, antiviral, and mucolytic agent. The thyroid gland uses iodine on a daily basis. Iodine is needed for the production of thyroid hormones.

Iron. Iron and other minerals play an important role in hormone synthesis. Optimal levels of ferritin (storage iron) are 100 ng/ml. If you are a menstruating woman then your ferritin levels should be at least 130 ng/ml since you lose iron every month when you menstruate. High levels of ferritin increase your risk of heart disease, so ask your health care provider if you need to take iron.

Magnesium. There is a direct link between magnesium and a healthy thyroid and heart related conditions, however, a magnesium deficiency is difficult to test for. You can boost your magnesium intake by eating a well-balanced diet which includes dark, leafy vegetables, seeds and nuts, and eliminate caffeine from your diet. Magnesium supplements, such as a pill or magnesium oil, should be taken with caution since they may interact with certain medications. If you are taking any medications check with your health care provider to see if there is a negative interaction.

Selenium. One study looked at patients that were critically ill and showed that supplementation with selenium normalized thyroid lab results. Adding one or two Brazil nuts or garlic to your diet every day can help to provide you with the needed selenium supplementation. You can get toxic with the use of selenium; therefore see your doctor or other health care provider before starting high doses of selenium.

Vitamin B2. Making sure you are getting enough vitamin B2 is necessary in regulating thyroid enzymes and maintaining healthy thyroid function. Eating almonds, eggs in moderation, cashews, salmon, and broccoli help to boost your B2 levels.

Vitamin B3. Vitamin B3 is instrumental in building a strong immune system, and the cause of an underactive thyroid has often been associated with a weak immune system. For a mild vitamin B3 deficiency 50 to 100 mg per day is recommended.

Vitamin D. Vitamin D is key in keeping your bones strong; however research suggests that low levels of vitamin D may have an effect on the thyroid working properly, as well as your immune system. See your health care provider to have her vitamin D levels measured to determine your exact dose.

Zinc. Zinc supplementation has been shown to help with optimal thyroid hormone metabolism. Eating a healthy diet and zinc supplements can be taken to treat a zinc deficiency. Taking too much zinc can cause toxicity. Zinc deficiency in humans can result from a reduced dietary intake and an inadequate absorption of the mineral.

Thyroid Hormone Replacement Therapy

When you consider thyroid hormone replacement, it is important to look at how the thyroid hormone is metabolized in the body. The body requires about 50 mg per year of iodine. About 70 percent of the T4 secreted daily is deiodinated to yield T3 and reverse T3 in equal parts. Eighty percent of circulating T3 comes from the peripheral monodeionization of T4 at the thyrosol ring which occurs in the liver, kidney, and other tissues. Circulating reverse T3 is made the same way. Thyroid hormone is also metabolized in other pathways. It can be conjugated with glucuronate or sulfate and then excreted in the bile or it can be decarboxylated. Twenty percent to 40 percent of T4 is subsequently eliminated in the stool.

Studies have shown that most patients do better, if they need thyroid replacement, to have both T3 and T4 replaced. One study of 89 patients with hypothyroidism that were previously treated with T4 alone was compared to a group of people with low thyroid function that were not treated with T4. The symptoms of the patients already on T4 were not any different from the people who were untreated. In fact, intracellular thyroid hormone receptors have a high affinity for T3. Ninety percent of the thyroid hormone molecules that bind with the receptors are T3 and 10 percent are T4. Other studies have verified that most individuals have less symptoms if they are prescribed both T3 and T4. In another study the lab results were not better, but the patients felt better if they took both T3 and T4.

There are different ways to take thyroid hormone replacement. They are all a prescription. You can take T4 alone, take T3 alone, or take both T4 and T3 which is commonly prescribed as desiccated thyroid, porcine (from a pig). If you have Hashimoto's thyroiditis (see page 36), some studies in the medical literature suggest that porcine thyroid replacement may not be the best form to take. This problem can be solved by your doctor prescribing non-porcine thyroid hormone which is compounded.

The following are common combined thyroid hormones that are available in North America as a prescription. Most of them are close to four parts T4 to one part T3:

- Armour thyroid (porcine) (ratio: T4 4 to T3 1)

- Euthroid (ratio: T4 4 to T3 1)

- Liotrix (ratio: T4 4 to T3 1)

- S-P-T (pork thyroid suspended in soybean oil)

- Thyrar (bovine)

- Thyroid Strong (ratio: T4 3.1 to T3 1)

- Thyroid USP (ratio: T4 4.2 to T3 1)

- Thyrolar (ratio: T4 to T3 1)

Next are the most common prescription T4 available in North America. All are immediate release and may contain lactose which can interfere with thyroid hormone absorption. Absorption can vary from 48 to 80 percent:

- Eltroxin
- Levothyroid
- Levoxyl
- Synthroid

Lastly are the most common T3 medications available in North America, all of which are immediate release:

- Cytomel
- Liothyronine sodium (generic)
- Triostat (injectable)

Compounded thyroid medication is made by a compounding pharmacy that is specially trained to make compounded medications. The advantage to having your thyroid hormone compounded is that you then can have the ratio of your T4 and T3 be any ratio that you want it to be. Four to one may not be the best ratio for you. In other words, compounded prescription thyroid medication is customized to your own needs. It is personalized. One size does not fit all patients. Also, you are getting no fillers and the physician who writes your prescription for compounded thyroid hormone can also add selenium, chromium, zinc, iodine, or other nutrients if needed.

It is crucial that when you are started on thyroid medication that you have your thyroid levels re-measured in six weeks. Once you have an optimal dosage schedule then your thyroid level should be re-measured every six months. There are things that can change your dose of thyroid medication, such as weight gain or weight loss. The amount of stress that you have may also affect your thyroid dosage.

OUTCOME (PROGNOSIS)

Once the source of the hypothyroidism has been identified and eliminated, any further damage to the thyroid gland should stop. However, normally, patients are put on a combination of T3 and T4 hormone for the rest of their lives to normalize their thyroid hormone level. Once done, all the symptoms and signs of hypothyroidism should be reversed.

HASHIMOTO'S THYROIDITIS (HT)

Hashimoto's thyroiditis, also called Hashimoto's disease, chronic lymphocytic thyroiditis, and autoimmune thyroiditis, is an autoimmune condition. Normally your immune system is designed to attack disease-causing
invaders such as bacteria or a virus, however, under certain conditions, it
can attack the thyroid gland, which can result in an inflammation of the
thyroid called Hashimoto's thyroiditis. As the tissues of the gland become
inflamed, the thyroid produces less hormones, interfering with the body's
normal metabolism. The disease begins slowly and may go undetected for
months or even years.

HT is the most common cause of hypothyroidism. It can result from
inherited genetic and environmental factors which often lead to a low
functioning thyroid. It most often affects middle-aged women, although
it can also affect men and teenagers. Generally, the symptoms and signs
resemble those of hypothyroidism. The disease progresses slowly and
causes a chronic thyroid disorder.

RISK FACTORS

The flare-up of antibodies that are at the root cause of Hashimoto's thyroiditis can be initiated for any number of reasons. The following factors
may indicate if an individual is at a higher risk:

Age

The signs of HT usually present between the ages of 30 and 50. The disease can occur in children, teens, and young women.

Gender

As with most thyroid related diseases, women are more prone to develop
HT than men.

Genetics

Recent research has shown a significant role of heredity in the development of autoimmune thyroid disease or Hashimoto's thyroiditis. In addition, other autoimmune- prone genes may trigger this condition as well.
However, it may require one or more environmental factors, as listed
below, to initiate this condition.

CAUSES

There are a number of conditions that may trigger HT. These include the following:

Environmental Exposure

There are a number of chemicals that may lead to the development of HT as well as other forms of autoimmune diseases. These include perchlorate, fluoride, lithium, mercury, bisphenol A, and Teflon.

Excessive Iodine

A diet heavy in foods containing iodine, taking iodine supplements, and/or taking drugs containing large amounts of iodine can trigger HT.

Pregnancy

Pregnancy creates great hormonal changes in a woman's body. Sometimes this can result in some form of thyroid dysfunction during or after pregnancy. Statistics indicate that approximately 20 percent of the women who have thyroid issues during pregnancy will develop HT in later years.

Radiation Exposure

While less common, research has shown that being exposed to large amounts of radiation can bring on autoimmune thyroid diseases.

SIGNS AND SYMPTOMS

The signs and symptoms of Hashimoto's thyroiditis are the same as those for hypothyroidism. (See page 24.)

DIAGNOSIS

Early diagnosis of Hashimoto's thyroiditis isn't always easy. Most people with an underactive thyroid aren't aware that they have this condition. They may suffer a number of symptoms without realizing they have a thyroid problem. There are several tests to indicate whether or not it may be HT. The key factor is to determine if the hypothyroidism is being caused by an autoimmune reaction.

Self-Awareness

As you have seen on page 24, there are many signs and symptoms associated with the underproduction of thyroid hormones. Low levels of thyroid hormones can cause many health issues to occur. If you see that you suffer from a number of these problems, you can conduct a simple home test to see if there is a possibility of you having this condition.

Home Testing

If you are experiencing specific signs or symptoms that indicate you may have an underactive thyroid (see page 24), you can administer a safe and simple home test (see inset on page 28). You can determine the possibility of any potential thyroid dysfunction on your own, at your home, by measuring your basal temperature. Although this test is obviously not an official diagnosis of a thyroid dysfunction, it can give you some indication that you need to follow up with your physician for further testing to be administered.

Consult With Your Doctor

If you feel a problem does exist, it is very important that you see your health care provider for an evaluation of your thyroid gland; and, that you have a complete workup done and not a partial workup.

Clinical Evaluation

Your physician will perform a complete physical exam of the gland, where he/she palpates your thyroid to determine if there are any lumps, nodules, growths (goiters), or masses. In addition, he/she will be checking the thyroid's size, and if it is solid and firmly fixed in place.

Blood Tests

The blood test is the most common test, and plays an important role in diagnosing thyroid disease and treating thyroid conditions. A number of blood tests will be done in order to determine if you are suffering from hypothyroidism. Your physician will be evaluating your TSH, free T4, freeT3, rt3 (reverse T3), and thyroid antibodies (see Table 1.2 on page 12).

Thyroid binding globulin (TBG) can also be measured (see page 13). This is the amount of stored hormone. It is produced by the liver and is affected by illness, liver disease, and some medications. Sometimes estrogens can raise TBG so this is another test that your doctor may order. Your health care provider may also order thyroid releasing hormone (TRH), also called thyrotropin-releasing factor (TRF), which is a hormone that stimulates the release of thyroid stimulating hormone (TSH) and prolactin from the pituitary (see page 13).

In addition, with HT, the person's high antibody level compared to a lowered level of thyroid hormones will indicate the presence of autoimmune problem. Likewise, it is not as common but you can have normal levels of TSH, free T3, and free T4 with positive antibodies and you would still have HT.

Fine Needle Aspiration (FNA)

Fine needle aspiration is a type of biopsy procedure that is commonly performed to detect or rule out cancer cells in the thyroid. It is commonly performed on swellings or lumps found in the thyroid. The fine needle aspiration can identify the type of cells contained in the abnormal tissue or fluid. (See Chapter 3, page 49.)

Imaging Tests

Laboratory tests may not be enough to diagnosis thyroid dysfunction. Sometimes more tests are ordered. Imaging tests are administered for a diagnosis of various thyroid disorders. The following are some other tests that may be performed:

- Iodine Uptake Scan: to measure the absorption of iodine in the thyroid.

- Thyroid Scan: a radioisoptope is administered, usually given with the iodine uptake. Cells that do not absorb iodine will appear "cold" (lighter on the scan), a cell absorbing too much iodine will appear "hot" (darker).

- Thyroid Ultrasound: high frequency sound waves provide an image of the thyroid gland. It aids in performing fine need biopsies.

TREATMENT OF HASHIMOTO'S THYROIDITIS

Once a diagnosis of HT has been confirmed there are a number of therapies available to treat the condition detailed on page 36. With HT, patients should seek to reduce the level of their body's autoimmune response. A safe way to do this can be to avoid any foods that may contribute to this process. Consider going on a **detox** diet that pulls out inflammatory foods which may alleviate **thyroid** symptoms (see Detoxification section on page 30). Also avoiding gluten, foods you are allergic to, and having optimal gastrointestinal function may decrease or resolve your symptoms. (See Chapter 9 on Thyroid Hormones and Digestive Health, page 145.) Furthermore, studies have shown that supplementing with selenium at a dose of 200 mcg decreased TPO antibodies and normalized the levels in some of the patients. Please check with your health care provider before starting selenium.

OUTCOME (PROGNOSIS)

While Hashimoto's thyroiditis cannot be cured, it can be well managed. By treating HT with thyroid hormones, normal thyroid hormone levels can be restored reversing any of its signs and symptoms. In addition, by staying away from foods that may increase inflammation in your body, you may avoid worsening your body's immune response.

If you are a woman of childbearing age with HT, you may have trouble conceiving, so talk to your doctor when planning for a pregnancy.

DISORDERS CAUSED BY OR ASSOCIATED WITH HYPOTHYROIDISM

There are many diseases and conditions that have been associated with hypothyroidism. Depression has been strongly associated with hypothyroidism, as have heart disease and memory loss. These disease processes are covered in separate chapters in this book.

Ankylosing Spondylitis (AS)

Ankylosing spondylitis is a kind of chronic rheumatic disease that affects the spine. The spine's vertebrae may fuse together, causing pain and stiffness from the neck down to the lower back. Eventually it may result in a stooped-over posture. This condition affects men two to three times more commonly than women. The inflammation that occurs in ankylosing spondylitis has been a subject of research. This inflammatory process has been linked in some individuals with low functioning thyroid and the activation of the body's immune system.

Attention Deficit Hyperactivity Disorder

Attention Deficit Hyperactivity Disorder is a condition characterized by impulsive symptoms, inattention, being easily distracted, forgetfulness, and hyperactivity that affects every day functioning. Some studies have shown that ADHD may be related to thyroid dysfunction. They found that increased levels of TSH correlated with an inability to sustain one's attention.

Chronic Fatigue Syndrome (CFS)

Chronic fatigue syndrome has been associated with an underactive thyroid, however it is very often misdiagnosed. When diagnosed properly, the majority of cases are women in the age bracket of 25 to 45 years old. CFS is a medical condition where you suffer from long-term fatigue that is not due to exertion and this condition puts limitations on your ability to carry out normal daily activities. Research has indicated that a relationship may exists between CFS and thyroid autoimmunity. These studies suggest that the immune system may be chronically active which would explain the fatigue and lack of energy you experience.

Fibromyalgia (FMS)

Fibromyalgia is an arthritic related condition characterized by widespread musculoskeletal pain, soreness, and tenderness that rarely disappears. It is one of the most common chronic pain conditions also affecting women more than men. The most common symptoms of FMS mimic low thyroid symptoms and is therefore often misdiagnosed. Some experts suggest that FMS is also related to the immune dysfunction and others suggest that it is an indication of an underactive metabolism, a low thyroid disorder, and/or a dysfunction of the mitochondria (the energy producing cells of the body).

Insulin Sensitivity or Insulin Resistance

Insulin sensitivity indicates that the body has become resistant to the effects of insulin and can eventually lead to type II diabetes. One study showed that lower TSH and higher T4 levels are associated with improved insulin sensitivity, higher HDL, and better endothelial (pertaining to inner lining of blood vessels) function.

Weight Gain

Thyroid hormones regulate your metabolism including your basal metabolic rate. Therefore, hypothyroidism may be the hidden cause of a weight problem. Thyroid hormones can have a major effect on your waistline. Low thyroid function can add pounds to your body while making it difficult to lose weight. This means that even if you watch what you eat, your body is less able to convert calories into energy. Those unused calories end up causing you to gain weight. Slowly, over time, you can gain 10 to 15 pounds without even realizing it. Furthermore, the combination of reduced metabolism and other symptoms of hypothyroidism makes losing weight seem like a losing battle. The depression and insomnia so often caused by hypothyroidism increase your likelihood of indulging in foods that are high in less desirous carbohydrates and "bad" fats. Likewise, the fatigue associated with an underactive thyroid makes it harder for you to engage in the physical activity necessary to burn extra calories.

CONCLUSION

Optimal thyroid function requires adequate nutritional intake. It is also related to toxin exposure, other hormonal function, and medication usage. Likewise, as you have seen in this chapter, many factors determine optimal thyroid function including accurate measuring techniques. Most individuals that require thyroid replacement benefit from both T3 and T4 to optimize thyroid function and consequently improve overall health. In the next chapter you will learn about the symptoms, causes, diagnoses, and treatments for hyperthyroidism; when the thyroid makes too much thyroid hormone.

3

Hyperthyroidism

As a general definition, hyperthyroidism usually refers to the over-production of thyroid hormones in the body. However, when you read medical texts, there are two terms that are associated with the over production of thyroid hormones. They are hyperthyroidism and thyrotoxicosis, and while they both refer to the production of too much thyroid hormone in your body, they are two distinctly different conditions.

The term hyperthyroidism refers to disorders that result from long-term overproduction and release of hormones by the thyroid gland. For individuals with hyperthyroidism, the greater number of symptoms can be very subtle and take several weeks to months to be noticed. This occurs because the slight elevation in thyroid hormones is so small that the patient may not notice or put off going to the doctor. Hyperthyroidism is a long-term condition.

On the other hand, thyrotoxicosis refers to an excessive thyroid hormone production that is caused by a physiologically-based change in the gland. For example, as will be discussed later, it can be caused by an inflamed or damaged thyroid gland, or by taking or stopping certain drugs. People that have thyrotoxicosis can usually pinpoint the date that their symptoms began and seek medical attention immediately.

With a normally functioning thyroid gland, hormones are released into the blood stream over a 30 to 60 day period. In the case of thyrotoxicosis, hormones are released over a shorter period of time, such as a few days or a couple of weeks. This is referred to as a transient hormone excess state. Should thyrotoxicosis occur within an even shorter period of time, this condition is referred to as a thyroid storm or thyroid crisis. It should be considered an emergency situation and be treated immediately. If left untreated, it can lead to death.

Because hyperthyroidism is sometimes used as an overall term for the overproduction of thyroid hormones, thyrotoxicosis may be considered a category of hyperthyroidism. This can be confusing because the treatments for thyrotoxicosis may be very different from those offered for other hyperthyroid-related disorders. There are a number of disorders caused by or associated with hyperthyroidism and/or thyrotoxicosis. These include the following:

- Exogenous causes
- Factitious hyperthyroidism (seen in patients trying to lose weight)
- Latrogenic hyperthyroidism
- Iodine-induced hyperthyroidism (Jod-Basdow disease)
- Grave's disease (an autoimmune process)

- Hashimoto's thyroiditis in the early stages
- Painless thyroiditis
- Radiation thyroiditis
- Subacute thyroiditis
- Thyroiditis
- Toxic goiters
- Multinodular goiter
- Toxic adenomas

HYPERTHYROIDISM

As we see, there are a number of forms hyperthyroidism can take. In order to establish if it is hyperthyroidism, we need to be able to identify the condition and know what our options are. The following section is designed to provide you with such information.

RISK FACTORS

There are a number of risk factors that can increase the possibility of developing hyperthyroidism. The following elements may indicate if an individual is at increased risk:

Age

Hyperthyroidism can occur at any age, but it is more common in people 60 years old or older. On the other hand, Graves' disease usually occurs between the ages of 20 and 40.

Gender

In general, women are more likely to develop hyperthyroidism than men. In regard to Graves' disease, there are eight females for every one male with this specific disease.

Genetics

Statistics strongly indicate that genetics plays a role in a person's predisposition to develop hyperthyroidism. While there is no evidence that only one gene is to blame, it is more likely that the presence of several specific genes increase the incidence of hyperthyroidism. However in order to turn these genes on, it may require one or more triggers, as listed below, to initiate this condition.

Ethnicity

Statistically, the Japanese appear to be at greater risk for hyperthyroidism than other people. This may be attributed to either genetics or a diet high in iodine rich foods.

CAUSES OF HYPERTHYROIDISM

When the thyroid is diseased it may produce and release too much thyroid hormone. A number of conditions may be the cause for the overproduction of the thyroid hormone, including:

Emotional and Physical Stress

Recent stress may be a precipitating factor in the development of hyperthyroidism, especially in the class of Graves' disease. The most common precipitating factor is the "actual or threatened" separation from an individual upon whom the patient is emotionally dependent.

Environmental Toxic Exposure

Studies done on lab animals showed that exposure to toxic levels of cadmium and/or mercury increased the risk of developing hyperthyroidism.

Excess Dietary Iodine Supplementation

Iodine excess may be a problem particularly in people that take iodine without having their iodine levels measured. Common sources of iodine are iodinized salt, betadine washes, and iodine-containing medications, such as amiodarone and radiographic dyes.

A large study looked at the rate of Graves' disease in a population that was required to consume iodized salt. The rate of thyrotoxicosis and Graves' disease was higher throughout the entire study time. The increase in rate included both nodular and diffuse goiters. The conclusion of the study was that iodine supplementation in a group of people that were iodine-sufficient can increase the risk of developing thyrotoxicosis in susceptible people. However, it is important to point out that not having enough iodine can also lead to additional thyroid issues. Make sure to talk to your healthcare provider regarding your own situation, and keep track of your iodine levels when your test results come in.

Existing Autoimmune Diseases

For those people with preexisting immune system disorders, such as type 1 diabetes or rheumatoid arthritis, studies have shown there is an increased risk of developing Graves' disease.

Infections

Viral and bacterial infections have been reported in a large percentage of patients with Graves' disease. Studies indicate that a number of these pathogens can trigger the body's immune system to create antibodies; and it is in the body's natural response that a specific antibody may attach itself to the thyroid cells to overproduce hormones.

Medications

Some medications, such as amiodarone, lithium, interferon-alpha, IL-2, and GM-CSF (granulocyte-macrophage colony-stimulating factor), can cause an inflammation of the thyroid gland which in turn can cause an overproduction of thyroid hormones. In addition, taking too much thyroid hormone can lead to hyperthyroidism.

Pregnancy and Recent Childbirth

For women going through pregnancy, there are a number of hormonal changes that their bodies experience. This includes increases in progesterone, estrogen, oxytocin, prolactin, and relaxin—any of these hormones could trigger the development of Graves' disease.

Smoking

Smoking has a significant impact on thyroid function interfering with the thyroid's ability to absorb iodine. Oddly enough, in some individuals it can result in an excess amount of thyroid hormone production, and in others, a reduction.

Thyroid Nodules (Toxic Adenoma, Toxic Multinodular Goiter, Plummer's Disease)

A benign growth or nodule that has walled itself off from the rest of the gland may cause an enlargement of the thyroid. When this happens the gland may produce an excess amount of the hormone T4 which will then enter into the blood.

Thyroiditis (Inflamed Thyroid Gland)

The thyroid gland can become inflamed for a variety of reasons. This inflammation can cause the gland to increase in size and to produce excess amounts of thyroid hormone which will then enter into the bloodstream.

SIGNS AND SYMPTOMS

The following are the most common signs and symptoms of hyperthyroidism and/or thyrotoxicosis. The progression of these individual symptoms, however, may also differ from one individual to another. It is also important to keep in mind that many of these symptoms can be caused by other underlying problems.

Early Symptoms

❑ Anxiety, nervousness, and irritability

❑ Brittle fingernails

❑ Breast enlargement in men (rare)

❑ Bulging eyes (exophthalmia)

❑ Constipation

❑ Diarrhea and/or an increase in bowel movements

❑ Difficulty in managing diabetes

❑ Elevated heart rate (tachycardia) and/or chest pain

❑ Erectile dysfunction or reduced sexual urges

❑ Eyelid retraction, puffy eyelids, reddening around the eyes, pressure on the eyes, and irritation of the eyes as well as double vision (Graves' thyroid eye disease)

❑ Goiter (enlargement of the thyroid gland)

❑ Heart palpitations (sensation heart is pounding)

❑ Heat or cold intolerance

❑ Muscle weakness

❑ Personality or psychological changes

❑ Perspiring profusely (diaphoresis)

❑ Separation of nail from the nail bed (onycholysis)

❑ Shortness of breath

❑ Skin changes

❑ Slight trembling of the hands or fingers

❑ Weight change (weight loss or gain)

Late Symptoms

❑ Decreased ability to hear

❑ Hoarseness

❑ Lumpy thickening and reddening of the skin, usually on the shins or tops of the feet (Graves' dermopathy)

❑ Menstrual disorders

❑ Puffy face, hands, and feet

❑ Slow speech

❑ Thinning eyebrow hair

Most commonly, younger patients tend to show symptoms of sympathetic activation—that is, the fight or flight response—which brings on anxiety, hyperactivity, and tremors. With patients over 60, the symptoms may more frequently involve cardiovascular related issues which need to be carefully monitored.

TESTING FOR HYPERTHYROIDISM

If you are experiencing any of the symptoms associated with hyperthyroidism, there are a number of tests available to determine whether you have hyperthyroidism or thyrotoxicosis.

Physical Examination

Normally, a physician can see some of the more pronounced signs, such goiters, thyroid enlargement, or signs of tremors, which can indicate hyperthyroidism.

Blood Tests

In a standard blood test, there is usually an increase in the level of thyroid hormones (T3 and T4). There is also a compensatory decrease in the level of the thyroid-stimulating hormone (TSH) since the thyroid is now being stimulated by an antibody, TSH production would naturally drop. In another specialized blood test, the level of the thyroid peroxidase antibody (TPO) is measured. This may indicate that there is an autoimmune disorder present. However since 5 percent to 10 percent of healthy individuals test positive for TPO, the results of this antibody test may not be conclusive. If the tests all come back within a normal range, these blood tests can at least rule out hyperthyroidism.

Fine Needle Aspiration (FNA)

If a node is found, a fine-needle aspiration is done. The skin above the node is numbed, and a thin needle is inserted into the node to remove cells and fluid for review. These samples are then sent to a laboratory where a pathologist examines them under a microscope to determine the exact nature of the cells. The pathologist writes up a report on the findings and sends back the report to the ordering physician.

While the FNA is designed to determine if the cells are benign or cancerous, up to 30 percent of the FNA biopsies may be inconclusive. When this happens a blood test may be able to provide an answer. However, should it not, traditionally, surgery is the next step to determine if the node is benign or cancerous. Recently, however, a new personalized genetic test has been developed to provide an answer based on the initial FNA biopsy which can help prevent unnecessary surgeries. (See Personalized Genetic Test below.)

Personalized Genetic Tests

Beyond just testing for inherited thyroid cancer-prone genes, there are new personalized genetic tests available which may be able to rule out whether the cells taken from a FNA procedure are benign or malignant. Additionally, the tests may also be able to determine how aggressive a cancerous thyroid cell may be. These tests are based upon molecular identification. The results of such tests can enable a surgeon to determine how extensive a surgery is needed or if one is required at all. (See Chapter 10 for more on Thyroid Cancer, page 157.)

Radioactive Iodine Uptake (RAIU)

A radioactive iodine uptake test (RAIU) is designed to measure the amount of iodine your thyroid absorbs and determine whether all or only part of the thyroid is overactive. The amount of radioactive tracer your thyroid absorbs determines if your thyroid function is normal or abnormal. A high uptake of iodine tracer may mean you have hyperthyroidism.

Scan of Your Eye Area

In the case of Graves' disease, if the patient is showing either irritation around the eye and socket, or there is a bulging of the eyes, an ultrasound, magnetic resonance imaging (MRI), or computed tomography (CT) scan may be performed to determine the extent of impact the irritation has caused.

Thyroid Scan

A radioactive iodine tracer is injected into the vein in the arm or hand. You then lie on a table with a scanner that produces an image of your thyroid on a computer screen. The image can show whether parts of the thyroid gland are absorbing too much or too little of the radioactive iodine. This test may be given as part of a radioactive iodine uptake test. In that case, orally administered radioactive iodine is normally used to image the thyroid gland.

Based upon the patient's family history, risk factors, symptoms, and test results, the doctor will determine if the problem is hyperthyroidism.

TREATMENT OF HYPERTHYROIDISM

The treatment of choice for hyperthyroidism is governed by many factors. It depends on age, goiter size and association with nodular disease, existence of Grave's eye disease, standard of care in the area in which one lives, the personal preference of the treating physician, any other disease processes one may have, and of course the patient's choice. Treatment of thyroid storm is a medical emergency and must be treated immediately.

The goal of these treatments is to correct the overproduction of thyroid hormone. The following is a summary of common treatments for hyperthyroidism and thyrotoxicosis. Also see the chapters on Graves' disease and autoimmune thyroid disease for further therapies.

Anti-thyroid Medication

One of the first options offered is anti-thyroid medications. Anti-thyroid drugs are designed to interfere with the thyroid glands ability to produce hormones thereby decreasing hormone production. Unlike other treatments, once they are discontinued, they allow the thyroid to function as usual. Side effects many vary with each drug. These may include nausea, vomiting, heartburn, headache, rash, joint pain, loss of taste, liver failure, or a decrease in disease-fighting white blood cells. Pregnant women should always check with their doctor regarding when they can start on such medications. These drugs can usually be discontinued once a stable normal thyroid balance has been achieved with other therapies. These medications include the following:

Glucocorticoids. Glucocorticoids in high doses inhibit the peripheral conversion of T4 to T3. In the treatment of Grave's disease, glucocorticoids decrease T4 secretion by the thyroid gland. How effective this response is or how long it lasts is not known. Use of glucocorticoids is usually not suggested for hyperthyroidism and thyrotoxicosis unless there is major eye or skin involvement or if the patient is in thyroid storm. Short-term use only for these conditions is suggested.

Iodine and iodine-containing compounds. Pharmacologic doses of iodine as Lugol's solution or saturated solution of potassium iodide (SSKI) work by the following mechanisms:

- Decreases iodine transport into the thyroid

- Inhibits iodine organification and blocks the release of T4 and T3 from the thyroid gland

- Decreases the vascularity of the thyroid in Graves' disease

The effects are transient, lasting only a few days to weeks. Thyrotoxicosis may return and even worsen. Consequently, iodine therapy is used only short term in preparation for surgery after a normal state has been achieved and maintained with the use of thionamides. Iodine is also used to treat thyroid storm since it can inhibit thyroid hormone immediately.

Oral cholecystographic agents. Oral cholecystographnic agents (iodine containing radiocontrast agents), such as iopanoic acid and sodium ipodate, produce a rapid fall in thyroid hormones. They act by inhibition of the peripheral conversion of T4 to T3 and by prevention of thyroid hormone secretion because of the inorganic iodine that is released from the drug. Both iopanoic acid and sodium ipodate because of their rapid onset of action are very effective treatments for thyrotoxicosis. They are not effective for long-term treatment because of the escape of thyroid hormone synthesis from the blocking action of iodine. Furthermore, iopanoic acid and sodium ipodate provide a load of iodine to the thyroid which makes the using of radioactive iodine not feasible for weeks. Therefore, these drugs are best used for emergency situations for a rapid decrease in thyroid hormone production or prior to surgery.

Perchlorate. Perchlorate works by inhibiting the transport of iodine into the thyroid. Possible side effects include stomach irritation and aplastic anemia. These side effects are somewhat common, therefore it stops the use of perchlorate as treatment for hyperthyroidism/thyrotoxicosis long-term. Used in conjunction with thionamides, perchlorate has been used successfully for depleting the thyroidal iodine overload in amiodarone-induced hyperthyroidism.

Thionamides. There are three thionamides drugs, methimazole (MMI), carbimazole, and propylthiouracil (PTU) which are effective in their treatment of Graves'. Thionamides do not block the release of preformed thyroid hormone. Consequently it takes 1 to 6 weeks for the thyroid hormones that are already stored and the iodine that is stored to be depleted and the patient to have total relief of symptoms and normalization of thyroid studies. Large goiters with large deposits of thyroid hormone may show a delayed response to thionamides.

The main problem with the use of thionamides is that there is a high relapse rate of thyrotoxicosis when the medications are stopped. Recurrence rate is 50 to 80 percent depending on the length of follow-up. Most relapses occur within 3 to 6 months, but it can occur much later. Remission rates have decreased over the last decade, perhaps due to an increased iodine supply in the diet of the average American. Relapse to hyperthyroidism after treatment suggests that another form of treatment may be necessary. Some patients become hypothyroid after therapy.

Mild side effects have been reported in 1 to 15 percent of patients that take thionamides.

- Hives (urticaria)
- Itching (pruritus)
- Joint pain (arthralgias)
- Slightly elevated liver enzymes
- Skin rash

Severe side effects of thionamides are rare and require prompt discontinuation of the medication.

- Cholestatic necrotic hepatitis
- Decrease of white blood cells (agranulocytosis)
- Inflammation of blood vessels (vasculitis)
- Lupus-like syndrome
- Toxic hepatitis

Thionamides can be used prior to thyroid surgery, with radioactive iodine, or as primary treatment. Treatment is usually for 1 to 2 years and then stopped.

Beta blockers (B-Adrenergic Antagonist Drugs)

Beta blockers were originally designed to reduce blood pressure by blocking the effects of epinephrine, also called adrenaline. It does this by slowing down the number of heart beats per minute as well as opening up blocked vessels. This, in turn, reduces tachycardia, palpitations, tremor, and anxiety. The effects of beta blockers are fast, so it is important for use early on in the treatment of thyrotoxicosis. These drugs do not affect thyroid function, release, or synthesis. Beta blockers should not be used if you have asthma, emphysema, congestive heart failure, bradycardia (slow heart beat), hypotension (low blood pressure), COPD (chronic obstructive pulmonary disease), or Raynaud's phenomenon.

Radioactive Iodine Therapy

As discussed earlier, in order to function, the thyroid gland needs to absorb iodine on a daily basis. With this therapy, a radioactive form of iodine is orally taken by the patient. As the reactive iodine is absorbed, the low level radiation is enough to destroy the overactive thyroid cells causing the thyroid to shrink and to produce less hormones.

Because this treatment involves destroying thyroid cells, it will likely have an effect on the amount of thyroid hormones produced in the future. For that reason, a patient's thyroid hormone levels must be checked regularly, and that individual may require thyroid medication to make up for a drop in thyroid hormone production.

This treatment may not be effective in patients with large goiters; consequently several treatments may be needed. If you have a large goiter then surgery may be the therapy of choice. In the elderly, radioactive iodine is usually the treatment of choice. In women that are of childbearing age, they should delay pregnancy for 6 to 12 months after receiving radioactive iodine.

Surgery

Another possible treatment for hyperthyroidism is surgery. The goal of surgery is to decrease the excessive secretion of thyroid hormone and to prevent a relapse of thyrotoxicosis. For a long time, partial thyroidectomy was recommended. Recently, total thyroidectomy (the entire thyroid gland is removed) is more commonly performed. There is a higher rate of hypothyroidism associated with this procedure, but a lower rate of recurrence of hyperthyroidism.

Commonly your doctor will have you treated with thionamide, an anti-thyroid medication, to restore and maintain a normal thyroid state in preparation for surgery. Some surgeons may use inorganic iodine 10 days before surgery to induce the involution of the thyroid gland and decrease the vascularity which makes the surgery easier.

Surgery is the best choice for individuals that have a larger goiter, if cancer cannot be ruled out, if cancer is present, and if multiple cold nodules are not expected to respond with shrinkage to radioactive iodine.

Some of the possible side effects of surgery include: infection, bleeding, thyroid storm, injury to the recurrent laryngeal nerve, hypoparathyroidism, hypothyroidism, and hypocalcemia (low calcium level). With the partial or whole removal of your thyroid gland, a patient's levels of thyroid hormones must be carefully monitored.

NATURAL THERAPIES FOR HYPERTHYRODISM AND THYROTOXICOSIS

There are natural therapies for hyperthyroidism that have been shown to be clinically effective for mild disease. These may be used in conjunction with standard medical treatment. Before starting any, each natural option should be discussed with your health care provider.

Acupuncture

Acupuncture, the use of small needles strategically placed in the skin, has been used as a treatment in China for thousands of years. Studies in China have shown it effective in treating hyperthyroidism.

Cold packs

By placing ice packs over the thyroid gland, found at the base of your neck, three times a day you can reduce swelling. (See illustration on page 6.) The cold will also help slow down the function of the thyroid gland.

Diet

In treating your hyperthyroidism it is important to learn how to get as much nutrition as possible from your food and to learn to make good food choices.

Eat Foods That Are Good For You

Whole fruits, vegetables, and nuts head the list. In addition, a high protein diet has been shown to be effective against mild Graves' disease.

These foods contain goitrogens, a naturally-occurring chemical, which has been shown to prevent or make it more difficult to utilize iodine. In so doing, they block thyroid synthesis. These goitrogenic foods include:

- Almonds
- Broccoli
- Brussels sprouts
- Cabbage
- Cassava root
- Cauliflower

- Kohlrabi (a vegetable)
- Millet
- Mustard
- Peaches
- Peanuts

- Pine nuts
- Rapeseeds
- Rutabagas
- Soybeans
- Sweet potatoes
- Turnips

However, it is important to understand these foods cannot be reliably used in place of medications in the treatment of Graves' disease since their goitrogen content is low. Furthermore, cooking inactivates the goitrogens. Likewise, no substantial documentation is available to show that dietary goitrogens interfere with thyroid function if the patient has adequate levels of iodine.

Studies have shown that individuals with hyperthyroidism should eat foods that contain flavonoids since they decrease serum T4 and inhibit both the conversion of T4 to T3 and 5′deiodinase activity. Foods such as fruits and vegetables of yellow, orange, red, and purple color, such as blueberries, purple grapes, and cherries, contain flavonoids.

Limiting Your Food Choices

In addition to eating the right foods, you can minimize your hyperthyroid symptoms by avoiding certain foods.

Avoid caffeine. Caffeine can increase the severity of many Graves' disease symptoms, such as rapid heart rate, anxiety, and tremors. By eliminating products such as soda, coffee, tea, and chocolate from your diet, you can control some of these persistent issues.

Avoid foods that contain iodine. Foods that are high in iodine content, such as seaweeds, iodized salt, fish from the sea, and shellfish, should be avoided.

Avoid foods that you are allergic to. While it may be easy to identify foods and avoid the foods you are allergic to, some people have hidden food allergies that they may not be aware of (see the chapter on Thyroid

Hormones and Digestive Disorders). Many of these food allergies can aggravate symptoms of hyperthyroidism. Make sure you are aware of all the foods you may have allergies to.

Avoid processed foods. Cut down or stop consuming foods that are heavily processed, salted, and/or sugared. Also, make sure to consume foods low in iodine. Find a healthful diet that you can stick to.

Nutritional Supplements

Nutritional supplements may be helpful in the treatment of mild hyperthyroidism. Free radical injury occurs when the body is exposed to excess thyroid hormone. Furthermore, low antioxidant status has been found in patients with excess thyroid production. In fact, the degree of cell damage in Graves' disease has been shown to be directly correlated with the amount of oxidative stress that is present. Taking antioxidants such as vitamins A, C, and E have been shown to be helpful alone or in conjunction with medications.

Calcium Citrate. Calcium metabolism may be changed in hyperthyroidism where patients with Graves' disease have an increased risk of developing osteoporosis. Supplementing with calcium may be beneficial.

Coenzyme Q-10. Similar to a vitamin, this substance is a cofactor in the electron-transport chain which is the energy producing cycle in the body. Q-10 levels have been shown to be low in adults and children with hyperthyroidism. Studies have also shown that coenzyme Q-10 levels may return to normal after treatment of hyperthyroidism with conventional therapies. It may be helpful to supplement Q-10 in people with hyperthyroidism that have cardiac disease and also in individuals with long-standing uncorrected hyperthyroidism.

L-carnitine. This amino acid is used for the transport of long-chain fatty acids into the mitochondria. L-carnitine is an antagonist of thyroid hormone in peripheral tissues by inhibiting thyroid hormone entry into the nucleus of the cells. One study conducted over 6 months used carnitine in patients with hyperthyroidism. Patients taking L-carnitine improved their symptoms and liver profiles, but the patients that did not take L-carnitine were worse. The form of L-carnitine used should be L-carnitine alone or the acetic or propionic acid form and not the D-form. If you have compromised kidney function, you may not be able to take L-carnitine or the dose may need to be decreased, therefore contact your physician before taking L-carnitine.

Selenium. Subclinical (undetcted) hyperthyroidism may be due to low selenium intake. In fact, selenium deficiency alters the conversion of T4 to T3 in peripheral tissues such as the kidney and liver. One study found men fed low selenium diets that their serum T3 levels were increased. A medical trial showed that subjects with autoimmune thyroiditis were given 200 micrograms of selenium for 3 months and their antibodies decreased or resolved. Selenium is one of the supplements that should be considered as a therapy for mild hyperthyroidism in people that are not high in selenium or selenium toxic.

Vitamin A. Given in large doses this antioxidant has an inhibitory effect on the thyroid gland. Vitamin A supplementation has been shown to decrease the symptoms of Graves' disease. The exact mechanism by which vitamin A works is unknown. If you smoke then do not consider this therapy since large doses of vitamin A in smokers may be linked to an increased risk of developing lung cancer.

Vitamin C (Ascorbic acid). Animal studies have shown that thyroid hormone in excess can reduce ascorbic acid levels in the blood, liver, adrenal glands, thymus, and kidney. Studies in human trials in patients with hyperthyroidism have also shown an increase in excretion of ascorbic acid. Furthermore, trials have shown that the medications thiourea and thiouracil also lower ascorbic acid levels. Consequently supplementation with vitamin C is suggested in patients with hyperthyroidism. Supplementation does not affect the course of the disease, but it may decrease the symptoms and metabolic effects.

Vitamin E. The vitamin may be protective against the oxidative damage caused by hyperthyroidism. In an animal study, animals with hyperthyroidism were given vitamin E which helped to prevent the lipid peroxidation that is associated with hyperthyroidism. Human studies have shown that individuals with hyperthyroidism have low vitamin E levels. Consequently supplementation with vitamin E is suggested.

Zinc. Red blood cell zinc levels are lower in patients with hyperthyroidism since zinc needs are increased because of greater urinary zinc excretion in this disease process. Therapy with anti-thyroid medications has been shown to normalize RBC zinc levels 2 months after free T3 and free T4 were normalized.

Herbs

There are a number of botanical supplements that may be helpful in some patients with mild hyperthyroidism. It is always advisable to work with a trained professional when using such herbal supplementation.

Bugleweed. In fact, the German Commission E, Germany's equivalent to the FDA, recognizes the use of bugleweed for mild hyperthyroid conditions associated with the dysfunction of the nervous system based on pharmacologic studies. However, they also stated that in rare situations high dosages have resulted in thyroid enlargement and sudden discontinuation has increased disease symptoms.

Club moss. This herb has been studied for hyperthyroidism like bugleweed. Animal studies using club moss have shown its ability to block TSH activity at the receptor level, block the release of TSH from the thyroid, and suppress the iodine pump. It can also inhibit the peripheral T4-deiodination and conversion to T3.

Emblica officinalis. Animal studies using Emblica officinalis are promising. It was shown to reduce T3 and T4 concentrations by a significant amount. Human trials need to be done.

Flavonoids. There are also botanical medicines that contain flavonoids, such as hawthorne berry, astragalus, ginkgo biloba, licorice, and chamomile, that may be helpful for mild hyperthyroidism.

Ginger. It has been found that ginger has a positive effect on thyroid function. Ginger contains magnesium which has been proven to be a key factor in controlling thyroid disease. Since it aids in regulating inflammation, it is considered to also protect against thyroid conditions that are caused by inflammation. Ginger can be used in various ways. Fresh ginger root can be added when cooking or baking in the diced or powder form. In pill form, start with one capsule twice a day.

Lemon balm. This herb has calming effects on the nervous system and has been used since ancient times for this issue. In vitro studies have confirmed lemon balm's ability to block TSH receptors and inhibit both binding of bovine TSH to human thyroid tissue, and binding of autoantibodies in Graves' disease. Lemon balm has been used extensively in individuals with mild hyperthyroidism.

Motherwort. This is used traditionally to treat anxiety, depression, heart palpitations, and tachycardia. Therefore, it may be good for relief of symptoms of mild hyperthyroidism. It can be used with bugleweed. The German Commission E supports the use of motherwort for the treatment of cardiac disorders associated with anxiety and for the symptomatic relief of mild hyperthyroidism.

Turmeric. Turmeric is an herb that has been used for thousands of years. Like ginger, it can be beneficial in treating inflammation. It has anti-inflammatory properties which help to treat thyroid dysfunctions such as Graves' disease. You can add turmeric when cooking or it can be taken in capsule form. Follow dosage directions on the package.

OUTCOME (PROGNOSIS)

Once the source of the hyperthyroidism has been identified and eliminated, the overproduction of thyroid hormones should stop. However, as a result of a number of treatments, there can now be a permanent underproduction of thyroid hormones which can lead to hypothyroidism. (See page 17.) When this happens, patients are put on thyroid hormone for the remainder of their lives in order to normalize their thyroid hormone level. Once done, all the symptoms and signs of hypothyroidism should be reversed.

CONCLUSION

As you have seen in this chapter, hyperthyroidism is more common than you may have realized. It can go undetected for years appearing as any number of health issues. While it may not be immediately recognized for what it is, by understanding what causes it and what to look for, you can be your own best advocate. As you have seen in this chapter, there are many therapies, both conventional and natural, that have been found to be effective for hyperthyroidism.

While this chapter has provided you with a general overview of hyperthyroidism, there are more specific types of hyperthyroidism. We will examine these other forms in the next two chapters.

4

Graves' Disease

As seen in the previous chapter, there are a number of causes and treatments related to hyperthyroidism and thyrotoxicosis. On the other hand, Graves' disease is the most common form of hyperthyroidism. It is also known as diffuse toxic goiter and Flajani-Basedow-Graves disease. It represents 85 percent of all hyperthyroid cases. It is considered an autoimmune disease because of the way in which the body's immune system works against itself.

As we learned in Chapter 1, the pituitary gland produces thyroid stimulating hormone (TSH). TSH in turn triggers the thyroid gland into producing enough T3 and T4 hormones that the body requires. For any number of reasons, the body's immune system produces thyrotropin receptor antibody (TRAb) that acts in the same way TSH does, simulating the thyroid tissue to overproduce T3 and T4. In some cases the symptoms may be mild, while in other cases, the symptoms can be serious. Normally in Graves' disease, the entire thyroid gland becomes enlarged.

Unlike other forms of hyperthyroidism, Graves' disease can also affect the tissues and muscles surrounding the eyes and the eye socket inducing swelling and inflammation. This condition is called thyroid eye disease (TED) or opthalmopathy. Only 30 percent of Graves' patients show signs of TED. For those who do, the symptoms can range from mild to moderate to severe. While there are a number of therapies designed to reverse the overproduction of hormones brought about by Graves' disease, because TED involves the eyes, it may require other specialized treatments.

Grave's disease also occurs in 3 to 5 percent of people who have Myasthenia Gravis, a degenerative muscular disease.

RISK FACTORS

The flare-up of antibodies that are at the root cause of Graves' disease can be initiated by any number of reasons. The following factors may indicate if an individual is at a higher risk.

Age

The signs of Graves' disease usually present between the ages of 20 and 40.

Gender

For every one male patient with Graves' disease there are eight females. However, the ratio of patients that develop eye complications is equal in both men and women. Women with normal hormone levels of the estrogen but with an increased sensitivity to the estrogen have a higher prevalence of antibodies that may affect the thyroid.

Genetics

Statistics strongly indicate that genetics plays a role in a person's predisposition to develop Graves' disease. While there is no evidence that only one gene is too blame, it is more likely that the presence of several specific genes increase the incidencr of Graves' disease. Research has shown that Graves' disease is passed on from one generation to another as well as showing up in identical twins. However, it may require one or more triggers, as listed below, to initiate this condition.

Left-Handedness

Oddly enough, a study done by Wood and Cooper showed a statistically significant trend for left-handed people to be effected by Graves' disease.

CAUSES

Although Graves' disease has been studied for years, its causes remain unclear. There are, however, some conditions that are thought to be likely triggers.

Emotional and Physical Stress

Recent stress may be a precipitating factor in the development of Graves' disease. The most common precipitating factor is the actual or threatened separation from an individual upon whom the patient is emotionally dependent. Furthermore, studies now support the idea that Graves' disease often follows an emotional shock.

Existing Autoimmune Diseases

Graves' disease is caused by a breakdown in the body's disease-fighting immune system. For those people with preexisting immune system disorders, such as type 1 diabetes or rheumatoid arthritis, studies have shown that there is an increased risk of developing Graves' disease.

Infections

Viral and bacterial infections have been reported in a large percentage of patients with Graves' disease. Studies indicate that a number of these pathogens can trigger the body's immune system to create antibodies; and it is in the body's natural response that a specific antibody may attach itself to the thyroid cells to overproduce hormones.

Studies have reported an increase in the frequency of anti-influenza B virus antibodies found in patients with thyrotoxicosis. A large prevalence of circulating antibodies against the bacteria *Yersinia enterocolitica*, strain 0:3 have been seen in patients with Graves' disease. Also *Yersinia* antibodies have been found to interact with thyroid structures. Low-affinity binding sites for TSH have been found in other bacteria—*Leishmania* and *Mycoplasma.* Retroviral sequences or proteins have also been found in the thyroid gland of patients with Graves' disease. This may be due to a secondary infection.

Pregnancy and Recent Childbirth

For women going through pregnancy, there are a number of hormonal changes that their bodies experience. This includes increases in progesterone, estrogen, oxytocin, prolactin, and relaxin—any one of these or a combination of these hormones could trigger the development of Graves' disease.

Smoking

Studies showed a relatively small correlation between smoking and Graves' thyroid eye disease. There also appears to be an increase in symptoms when smoking is combined with drugs designed to stop the overproduction of thyroid hormones.

SIGNS AND SYMPTOMS

The following are the common signs and symptoms of Graves' disease. The progression of these, however, may also differ from one individual to another. It is also important to keep in mind that many of these symptoms can be caused by other underlying problems.

❏ Anxiety, nervousness, and irritability

❏ Breast enlargement in men (rare)

❏ Bulging eyes (exophthalmia)

❏ Chest pains and/or rapid or irregular heartbeat (palpitations)

❏ Difficulty in managing diabetes

❏ Erectile dysfunction or reduced sexual urges

❏ Eyelid retraction, puffy eyelids, reddening around the eyes, pressure on the eyes, and irritation of the eyes as well as double vision (Graves' thyroid eye disease)

❏ Goiter (enlargement of the thyroid gland)

❏ Heat intolerance

❏ Increase in bowel movements and/or diarrhea

❏ Lumpy thickening and reddening of the skin, usually on the shins or tops of the feet (Graves' dermopathy)

❏ Personality or psychological changes

❏ Perspiring profusely (diaphoresis)

❏ Shortness of breath

❏ Slight trembling of the hands or fingers

❏ Thinning hair

❏ Weight change (weight loss or gain)

If you think you have the onset of Graves' disease, review the tests listed below that are available to you, to evaluate your condition.

TESTING FOR GRAVES DISEASE

There are a number of tests available to determine whether you have Graves' disease or another potential form of hyperthyroidism.

Physical Examination

Normally, a physician can see some of the more pronounced signs, such as irritated or bulging eyes, thyroid enlargement, or signs of tremors which can indicate Graves' disease.

Blood Tests

In a standard blood test, there would be an increase in the level of thyroid hormones (T3 and T4) as would be expected with hyperthyroidism and there would be a decrease in the level of the thyroid-stimulating hormone (TSH). Because the thyroid is now being stimulated by an antibody, TSH production would naturally drop. In another specialized blood test, the level of the thyroid peroxidase antibody (TPO) is measured. This may indicate that there is an autoimmune disorder present. However, since 5 percent to 10 percent of healthy individuals test positive for TPO, the results of this antibody test may not be conclusive. If the tests all come back within a normal range, these blood tests can at least rule out Graves' disease.

Radioactive Iodine Uptake (RAIU)

A radioactive iodine uptake test (RAIU) is designed to measure the amount of iodine your thyroid absorbs and determine whether all or only part of the thyroid is overactive. The amount of radioactive tracer your thyroid absorbs determines if your thyroid function is normal or abnormal. A high uptake of iodine tracer may mean you have hyperthyroidism or Graves' disease.

Scan of the Area Around Your Eyes

If the patient is showing either irritation around the eye and eye socket, or there is a bulging of the eyes a number of scans can be ordered. Ultrasound, magnetic resonance imaging (MRI), or computed tomography (CT) scan may be performed to determine the extent of impact the irritation has caused.

Based upon the patient's family history, risk factors, symptoms, and test results, the doctor will determine if the problem is Graves' disease.

MEDICAL TREATMENTS

There are a number of the medical options available to combat Graves' disease. Each option should be considered in light of how far the Graves' disease has progressed.

Beta Blockers (B-Adrenergic Antagonist Drugs)

Beta blockers were originally designed to reduce blood pressure by blocking the effects of the hormone epinephrine, also called adrenaline. It does this by slowing down the number of heart beats per minute as well opening up blocked vessels. This, in turn, reduces tachycardia, palpitations, tremor, and anxiety. The effects of beta blockers are fast, so it is important for use early on in the treatment of Graves' disease. These drugs do not affect thyroid function, release, or synthesis. Beta blockers are not usually used alone for treatment of Grave's disease except for short time frames before and/or after radioactive therapy. Beta blockers should not be used if you have asthma, emphysema, congestive heart failure, bradycardia (slow heart beat), hypotension (low blood pressure), COPD (chronic obstructive pulmonary disease), or Raynaud's phenomenon.

Anti-thyroid Medication

One of the first options offered is anti-thyroid medications. Anti-thyroid drugs are designed to interfere with the thyroid gland's ability to produce hormones, thereby decreasing hormone production. Unlike other treatments, once they are discontinued, they allow the thyroid to function as usual. Side effects many vary with each drug. These may include nausea, vomiting, heartburn, headache, rash, joint pain, loss of taste, liver failure, or a decrease in disease-fighting white blood cells. Pregnant women should always check with their doctor regarding when they can start on such medications. These drugs can usually be discontinued once a stable normal thyroid balance has been achieved with other therapies. These medications include the following:

Glucocorticoids. Glucocorticoids in high doses inhibit the peripheral conversion of T4 to T3. In the treatment of Grave's disease, glucocorticoids decrease T4 secretion by the thyroid gland. How effective this response is or how long it lasts is not known. Use of glucocorticoids is usually not suggested for Graves' disease unless there is major eye or skin involvement or if the patient is in thyroid storm. Short-term use only for these conditions is suggested.

Iodine and iodine-containing compounds. Pharmacologic doses of iodine such as Lugol's solution or saturated solution of potassium iodide (SSKI) work by the following mechanisms:

- Decreases iodine transport into the thyroid

- Inhibits iodine organification and blocks the release of T4 and T3 from the thyroid gland

- Decreases the vascularity of the thyroid in Graves' disease

The effects are only transient lasting, only a few days to weeks. Thyrotoxicosis may return and even worsen. Consequently, iodine therapy is used only short term in preparation for surgery after a normal state has been achieved and maintained with the use of thionamides. Iodine is also used to treat thyroid storm since it can inhibit thyroid hormone immediately.

Oral cholecystographic agents. Oral cholecystographic agents (iodine containing radiocontrast agents), such as iopanoic acid and sodium ipodate, produce a rapid fall in thyroid hormones. They act by inhibition of the peripheral conversion of T4 to T3 and by prevention of thyroid hormone secretion because of the inorganic iodine that is released from the drug. Both iopanoic acid and sodium ipodate because of their rapid onset of action are very effective treatments for Graves' disease. They are not effective for long-term treatment because of the escape of thyroid hormone synthesis from the blocking action of iodine. Furthermore, iopanoic acid and sodium ipodate provide a load of iodine to the thyroid which makes the using of radioactive iodine not feasible for weeks. Therefore, these drugs are best used for emergency situations for a rapid decrease in thyroid hormone production or prior to surgery.

Perchlorate. Perchlorate works by inhibiting the transport of iodine into the thyroid. Possible side effects include stomach irritation and aplastic anemia. These side effects are somewhat common, therefore it stops the use of perchlorate as treatment for Graves' disease long-term. Used in conjunction with thionamides, perchlorate has been used successfully for depleting the thyroidal iodine overload in amiodarone-induced hyperthyroidism.

Thionamides. There are three thionamides drugs, methimazole (MMI), carbimazole, and propylthiouracil (PTU) which are effective in their treatment of Graves'. Thionamides do not block the release of preformed thyroid hormone. Consequently it takes 1 to 6 weeks for the thyroid hormones that are already stored and the iodine that is stored to be depleted and the patient to have total relief of symptoms and normalization of thyroid studies. Large goiters with large deposits of thyroid hormone may show a delayed response to thionamides.

The main problem with the use of thionamides is that there is a high relapse rate when the medications are stopped. Recurrence rate is 50 to 80 percent depending on the length of follow-up. Most relapses occur within 3 to 6 months, but can occur much later. Remission rates have decreased over the last decade, perhaps due to an increased iodine supply in the diet of the average American. Relapse after treatment suggests that another form of treatment may be necessary. Some patients become hypothyroid after therapy.

Mild side effects have been reported in 1 to 15 percent of patients that take thionamides, such as:

- Hives (urticaria)
- Itching (pruritus)
- Joint pain (arthralgias)

- Slightly elevated liver enzymes
- Skin rash

Severe side effects of thionamides are rare and require prompt discontinuation of the medication. These side effects include:

- Cholestatic necrotic hepatitis
- Decrease of white blood cells (agranulocytosis)

- Inflammation of blood vessels (vasculitis)
- Lupus-like syndrome
- Toxic hepatitis

Thionamides can be used prior to thyroid surgery, with radioactive iodine, or as primary treatment. Treatment is usually for 1 to 2 years and then stopped.

Radioactive Iodine Therapy

As discussed, in order to function, the thyroid gland needs to absorb iodine on a daily basis. With this therapy, a radioactive form of iodine is orally taken by the patient. As the reactive iodine is absorbed, the low level radiation is enough to destroy the overactive thyroid cells causing the thyroid to shrink and produce less hormones. The treatment is taken over several weeks. With the decrease in thyroid hormones, the symptoms of Graves' disease are lessened.

Unfortunately, in cases where there is eye muscle irritation, the outcome is more complicated. For patients with mild inflammation of the eye muscles, the results may be mild and temporary, however in cases that are moderate to severe this therapy is not recommended, nor is it recommended for women who are pregnant or nursing.

Because this treatment involves destroying thyroid cells, it will likely have an effect on the amount of thyroid hormones produced in the future. For that reason, an individual's thyroid hormone levels must be checked regularly, and that patient may require taking thyroid medication to make up for a drop in thyroid hormone production.

Surgery

In serious cases, surgically removing part or the whole thyroid gland may be considered. With the partial or whole removal of your thyroid gland, a patient's levels of thyroid hormones must be carefully monitored. If the entire or partial gland is removed, individuals will normally be required to take thyroid medication for the remainder of their lives.

Thyroid Eye Disease (TED) Treatments

For mild symptoms of TED, patients can use over-the-counter artificial tears during the day and lubricating gels at night to avoid corneal damage caused by exposure and for relief.

For moderate to severe symptoms, your doctor may recommend the following treatments:

Corrective lens. In cases of double vision because of Graves' disease, or as a side effect of surgery for Graves', glasses containing prism lens may be prescribed to normalize vision. The outcome of vision improvement may vary from patient to patient.

Corticosteroids. Treatment with corticosteroids, such as prednisone, will help reduce swelling behind your eyeballs. Side effects may include fluid retention, weight gain, elevated blood sugar levels, increased blood pressure, and mood swings.

Dry eyes. As soon as you begin to experience dry eyes or a sensation of grit or irritation in the eye, start to use artificial tears or eye drops to prevent any scratching of the cornea. Check with your doctor for a brand recommendation. You may also use eye covers at night to keep the eyes shut and prevent them from becoming dry.

Eyelid surgery. This procedure may be performed to restore the eyelid to an appropriate position allowing a patient to either close their eyes or to reduce sagging eyelid tissue to improve appearance.

Orbital decompression surgery. In this operation, the surgeon removes the bone between the eye socket and your sinuses, providing more room for the eyes to move back to their original position. This treatment should be considered when the pressure on the optic nerve may lead to blindness. Possible complications include double vision.

NATURAL TREATMENTS

While there are no natural short-cuts for treating Graves' disease, there are a number of natural treatment options to consider. These may be used in conjunction with standard medical treatment. Before starting any, each natural option should be discussed with your health care provider.

Acupuncture

Acupuncture, the use of small needles strategically placed in the skin, has been used as a treatment in China for thousands of years. Studies in China have shown it effective in treating Graves' disease.

Cold Packs

By placing ice packs over the thyroid gland, found at the base of your neck, three times a day you can reduce swelling. The cold will also help slow down the function of the thyroid gland.

Diet

Eat foods that are good for you. Whole fruits, vegetables, and nuts head the list. In addition, a high protein diet has been shown to be mildly effective against mild Graves' disease. These foods contain goitrogens, a naturally-occurring chemical, which has been shown to prevent or make it more difficult for utilization of iodine. In so doing, they block thyroid synthesis. These goitrogenic foods include:

- Almonds
- Broccoli
- Brussels sprouts
- Cabbage
- Cassava root
- Cauliflower

- Kohlrabi
- Millet
- Mustard
- Peaches
- Peanuts
- Pine nuts

- Rapeseeds
- Rutabagas
- Soybeans
- Sweet potatoes
- Turnip

However, it is important to understand these foods cannot be reliably used in place of medications in the treatment of Graves' disease since their goitrogen content is low. Furthermore, cooking inactivates the goitrogens. Likewise, no substantial documentation is available to show that dietary goitrogens interfere with thyroid function if the patient has adequate levels of iodine. Also foods that are high in iodine content, such as seaweeds, should be avoided.

Studies have shown that people should eat foods that contain flavonoids since they decrease serum T4 and inhibit both the conversion of T4 to T3 and 5'deiodinase activity. Food such as fruits and vegetables of yellow, orange, red, and purple color, such as blueberries, purple grapes, and cherries, contain flavonoids.

Exercise and Light-weight Training

While exercise is good for so many healthful reasons, when it comes to Graves' disease it can help in two ways. When the issue is weight gain, burning carbs through exercise can help keep pounds off. Secondly, with Graves' there is a tendency to have brittle bones. Light-weight training can strengthen bones as well as strengthen leg muscles for better balance and to prevent falls from occurring.

Limiting Your Food Choices

When treating Graves' disease you should avoid consuming any foods that will interfere with normal thyroid function.

Avoid caffeine. Caffeine can increase the severity of many Graves' disease symptoms, such as rapid heart rate, anxiety, and tremors. By eliminating products such as soda, coffee, tea, and chocolate from your diet, you can control some of these persistent issues.

Avoid foods that you are allergic to. While it may be easy to identify foods and avoid the foods you are allergic to, there are people who have hidden food allergies that they may not be aware of—from dairy (containing lactose) to soy to wheat (containing gluten) products. Many of these food allergies can aggravate Graves' symptoms. Make sure you are aware of all the foods you may be allergic to.

Avoid foods with high iodine content. It is wise to avoid foods containing a high level of iodine, such as sea vegetables, iodized salt, and some fish and seafood, since iodine can affect the overproduction of the thyroid hormones. In addition betadine washes, and iodine-containing medications, such as amiodarone and radiographic dyes, should be avoided if possible. Do not discontinue any medication without working with your physician. Iodine excess may be a problem particularly in people that take iodine without having their levels measured. The use of iodine in patients that have Graves' disease is unpredictable and it is not suggested for usage.

Avoid heavily processed foods. Cut down or stop consuming foods that are heavily processed, salted, and/or sugared. Also, make sure to consume foods low in iodine. Find a healthful diet that you can stick to.

Reducing Stress

Studies have shown that stress may trigger or worsen Graves' disease symptoms. By learning how to control stress in your life, you can avoid those stress-related hormones that may interfere in your healing process. Find the activity you enjoy most that you can relax doing—from taking long walks and hot baths to learning yoga exercises. This simple change in your life can make a difference.

Stop Smoking

Research has shown that smoking can increase the symptoms associated with Graves' disease—especially those who suffer from Graves' thyroid eye disease. In addition, it can affect the outcome of various thyroid treatments. Giving up smoking may not be easy, but it may be a lot easier to do knowing it's something that can help you beat the disease.

Nutritional Supplements

Another option for people with Graves' is taking nutritional supplements. However, taking nutritional supplements alone may not be enough to overcome this thyroid disease. There are a number of factors that should be considered when trying to improve your thyroid health, and taking certain nutritional supplements can be beneficial.

Calcium citrate. Calcium metabolism may be changed in hyperthyroidism where patients with Graves' disease have an increased risk of developing osteoporosis. Supplementing with calcium may be beneficial.

Coenzyme Q-10. Similar to a vitamin, this substance is a cofactor in the electron-transport chain which is the energy producing cycle in the body. Q-10 levels have been shown to be low in adults and children with hyperthyroidism. Studies have also shown that coenzyme Q-10 levels may return to normal after treatment of hyperthyroidism with conventional therapies. It may be helpful to supplement with Q-10 in people with Graves' disease that have cardiac disease and also in individuals with long-standing uncorrected hyperthyroidism.

L-carnitine. This amino acid is used for the transport of long-chain fatty acids into the mitochondria. L-carnitine is an antagonist of thyroid hormone in peripheral tissues by inhibiting thyroid hormone entry into the nucleus of the cells. One study conducted over 6 months used carnitine in patients with hyperthyroidism. Patients taking L-carnitine improved their symptoms and liver profiles, but the patients that did not take L-carnitine were worse. The form of L-carnitine used should be L-carnitine alone or the acetic or propionic acid form and not the D-form. Also L-carnitine is cleared through the kidneys so it should only be considered in individuals with normal kidney function.

Selenium. People with Graves' commonly have low selenium (a trace mineral) levels. In fact, selenium deficiency alters the conversion of T4 to T3 in peripheral tissues such as the kidney and liver. One study found men fed low selenium diets had their serum T3 levels increase. Selenium is one of the supplements that should be considered as a therapy for mild hyperthyroidism in people that are not high in selenium or selenium toxic. Eating Brazil nuts and other foods that are high in selenium is also helpful.

In a number of studies, it was found that a deficiency of selenium was found in a number of patients suffering from Graves' thyroid eye disease. When put on a daily dosage of 100 micrograms of selenium selenite twice daily for 6 months, there was an observable improvement of symptoms associated with mild TED. Additionally, the same amount of selenium taken by Graves' patients showed a significant decrease in their thyroid peroxidase antibody levels—one of the culprits that trigger the thyroid's overproduction of hormones.

Vitamin A. Given in large doses this antioxidant has an inhibitory effect on the thyroid gland. Vitamin A supplementation has been shown to decrease the symptoms of Graves' disease. The exact mechanism by which vitamin A works is unknown. If you smoke then do not consider this therapy since large doses of vitamin A in smokers may be linked to an increased risk of developing lung cancer.

Vitamin C (Ascorbic acid). Animal studies have shown that thyroid hormone in excess can reduce ascorbic acid levels in the serum, blood, liver, adrenal glands, thymus, and kidney. Studies in human trials in patients with hyperthyroidism have also shown an increase in excretion of ascorbic acid. Furthermore, trials have shown that the medications thiourea and thiouracil also lower ascorbic acid levels. Consequently, supplementation with vitamin C is suggested in patients with hyperthyroidism. Supplementation does not affect the course of the disease, but it may decrease the symptoms and metabolic effects.

Vitamin E. This vitamin may be protective against oxidative damage caused by Graves' disease. In an animal study, animals with hyperthyroidism were given vitamin E which helped to prevent the lipid peroxidation that is associated with hyperthyroidism. Human studies have shown that individuals with hyperthyroidism have low vitamin E levels. Consequently, supplementation with vitamin E is suggested.

Zinc. Red blood cell (RBC) zinc levels are lower in patients with Graves' disease since zinc needs are increased because of greater urinary zinc excretion in this disease process. Therapy with anti-thyroid medications has been shown to normalize RBC zinc levels 2 months after free T3 and free T4 were normalized.

Herbs

There are a number of botanical supplements that may be helpful in some patients with Graves' disease. It is always advisable to work with a trained professional when using such herbal supplementation.

Bugleweed. In fact, the German Commission E, Germany's equivalent to the FDA, recognizes the use of bugleweed for mild hyperthyroid conditions associated with the dysfunction of the nervous system based on pharmacologic studies. Activity is mediated by a reduction in TSH, T4, and inhibition of the conversion of T4 tp T3. Bugleweed also inhibits the recepter-binding and biological activity of Graves' immunoglobulins. However, be aware that in rare situations high dosages have resulted in thyroid enlargement and sudden discontinuation has increased disease symptoms.

Club moss. This herb has a long history of use for hyperthyroidism like bugleweed. Animal studies using club moss have shown its ability to block TSH activity at the receptor level, block the release of TSH from the thyroid, and suppress the iodine pump. It can also inhibit the peripheral T4-deiodination and conversion to T3.

Emblica officinalis. Animal studies using Emblica officinalis are promising. It was shown to reduce T3 and T4 concentrations by a significant amount. Human trials need to be done.

Ginger. It has been found that ginger has a positive effect on thyroid function. Ginger contains magnesium which has been proven to be a key factor in controlling thyroid disease. Since it aids in regulating inflammation, it is considered to also protect against thyroid conditions that are caused by inflammation. Ginger can be used in various ways. Fresh ginger root can be added when cooking or baking in the diced or powder form. In pill form, start with one capsule twice a day.

Lemon balm. Lemon balm has calming effects on the nervous system and has been used since ancient times for this issue. In vitro studies have confirmed lemon balm's ability to block TSH receptors and inhibit both binding of bovine TSH to human thyroid tissue and binding of auto-antibodies in Graves' disease. It is usually combined with bugleweed to treat Graves' disease. Studies show that this herb is helpful in lowering the production of thyroid hormones when given in injection form. More studies need to be done on the oral form.

Milk Thistle. Milk thistle is another natural therapy for the treatment of Graves' disease and is usually taken in supplement form for this purpose. It contains a flavonoid called silymarin that contains powerful antioxidant properties that are beneficial in the treatment of this disorder. It also may be helpful for treating eye problems caused by Graves' disease.

Motherwort. This is used traditionally to treat anxiety, depression, heart palpitations, and tachycardia. Therefore, it may be good for the relief of symptoms of Graves' disease. It can be used with bugleweed. The German Commission E supports the use of motherwort for the treatment of cardiac disorders associated with anxiety and for the symptomatic relief of mild hyperthyroidism.

Turmeric. Turmeric is an herb that has been used for thousands of years. Like ginger, it can be beneficial in treating inflammation. It has anti-inflammatory properties which help to treat thyroid dysfunctions such as Graves' disease. You can add turmeric when cooking or it can be taken in capsule form. Follow dosage directions on the package.

There are also botanical medicines that contain flavonoids, such as hawthorne berry, astragalus, ginkgo biloba, licorice, and chamomile that may be helpful therapies in Graves' disease.

OUTCOME (PROGNOSIS)

There are a number of factors that must be considered when treating Graves' disease: A patient's age, history of hyperthyroidism in their family, past and present health status, how serious their Graves' disease is, and their willingness to get better. For many patients with mild to moderate Graves' disease, their condition responds well to treatment. When they also have thyroid eye disease, both conditions must be treated together. Mild to moderate TED also responds well to treatments. Serious cases of TED may require additional eye surgery. Reversing the condition may take time, however the emphasis should be on maintaining a decent quality of life until it happens.

Thyroid surgery or radioactive iodine will usually cause an underactive thyroid (hypothyroidism). It is important to monitor your thyroid hormone levels to avoid the many effects of hypothyroidism. As long as you are getting the correct dosage of thyroid hormone replacement, you should be able to avoid the symptoms.

A number of the medical treatments described above may change your thyroid gland's normal hormone production. This may occur on a temporary basis or it can be permanent. When this happens, in order to keep your thyroid hormone level in balance, you will normally be required to take thyroid replacement. This may only be necessary until your thyroid is fully functioning or it may be necessary for the rest of your life.

CONCLUSION

As you have read, Graves' disease is the most common form of hyperthyroidism. Unfortunately, it can go undetected for years, masquerading as a host of other disorders. Once you have identified the problem as Graves', there is a good deal that can be done to reverse the condition. Of course, the earlier it is caught, the better the outcome. Still, knowing what your best options are and being able to participate in your return to health are important aspects of the healing process.

5

Thyroid Disorders Caused by or Associated with Hyperthyroidism and Thyrotoxicosis

As we have seen in the previous two chapters, there are a number of causes and treatments related to hyperthyroidism and thyrotoxicosis. In the same way there are a number of medical conditions that are created by or associated with hyperthyroidism and thyrotoxicosis. Many of these disorders come with their own set of symptoms, health issues, and treatments. If you believe that your may be suffering from an overproduction of thyroid hormones, this chapter should provide you with a basic understanding of the most common disorders related to this condition.

AUTONOMOUSLY FUNCTIONING THYROID NODULES (AFTN)

An autonomously functioning thyroid nodule (AFTN) is a well-defined mass of thyroid cells that grow either on the surface or within the thyroid gland. They may appear as either patchy areas, a single nodule, or as multiple nodules. When they appear as multiple nodules, this condition is referred to as Plummer's disease. These nodules are capable of producing and secreting thyroid hormone independent of stimulation by TSH. Because these nodules are capable of producing more thyroid hormones than the body requires, this condition can lead to hyperthyroidism.

There are two types of autonomously functioning thyroid nodules:

warm and hot. The term *warm* is given to nodules that do not produce sufficient amounts of hormones to disrupt the production of TSH. As a warm
nodule enlarges in size, it may begin to produce more thyroid hormones.
In addition, it may slow down the uptake activity of the surrounding thyroid tissue. When it produces an excess amount of thyroid hormone and
begins to affect the surrounding tissue, it is referred to as a *hot* nodule.
This condition can bring on hyperthyroidism. As it becomes bigger in
size, it can also be referred to as toxic.

Only a small number—5 to 10 percent—of solitary thyroid nodules are
toxic. This varies depending on the country the individual is from. For
example, the numbers are higher in Europe. The development of hyperthyroidism occurs mainly in nodules that are greater than 3 centimeters
with a minimal volume of 16 milliliters on an ultrasound of the thyroid.

It is important to also point out that just finding a nodule on the thyroid gland does not mean the growth is malignant. Each year there are
over 1.2 million patients who are diagnosed with thyroid nodules. Many
of these nodules are ruled out as benign using an ultrasound scan. Furthermore, of the 525,000 to 600,000 nodules that are biopsied every year,
only 10 percent are found to be malignant. (See Chapter 10 on page 157
for more information about malignant nodules.)

SIGNS AND SYMPTOMS

The signs and symptoms of patients with toxic adenoma or AFTN are the
same as they are for hyperthyroidism. (See Chapter 3, page 47.)

TESTS

There are a number of tests available to determine whether you have an
autonomously functioning thyroid nodule.

Physical Examination

Normally, a physician can see some of the more pronounced signs such a
lump in the neck, thyroid enlargement, or signs of tremors which can indicate hyperthyroidism.

Blood Tests

Unfortunately, measuring the level of the thyroid-stimulating hormone

(TSH) in your blood may not indicate whether or not you have AFTN. Because AFTN may not affect the TSH level, you will need an ultrasound scan to detect this condition.

Thyroid Ultrasound Scan

Sound waves are used to create a visual image of the thyroid. This is done when a small wand-like instrument is moved along the skin in front of the thyroid gland. The black and white image seen on a computer screen will show whether the node is composed of a solid mass of cells or a cyst containing blood or pus. If it is a solid node, further testing needs to be done to determine if the mass is benign or malignant.

Fine Needle Aspiration (FNA)

If a node is found, a fine-needle aspiration is taken. The skin above the node is numbed, and a thin needle is inserted into the node to remove cells and fluid for review. These samples are then sent to a laboratory where a pathologist examines them under a microscope to determine the exact nature of the cells. The pathologist writes up a report on his findings and sends back the report to the ordering physician.

TREATMENT

No treatment of a *hot* nodule is needed as long as you have normal thyroid function. Thyroid labs are usually repeated every 6 months since there is a concern for potential progression to hyperthyroidism. The possibility of a warm nodule being cancerous is there so it is evaluated the same way a *cold* nodule is. (A cold nodule is a thyroid nodule with a much lower uptake of radioactive iodine than the surrounding nodules during a radioactive iodine uptake scan, while a hot nodule shows an increase in radioactive uptake.) There are a number of effective treatments for AFTN. Your options may be based on the nature of your AFTN and the state of your health.

Surgery

If necessary, removing the node surgically may be a strong consideration. This therapy is very successful and only a small number of people become hypothyroid afterwards.

Radioactive Iodine Therapy (RAI)

With this therapy, a radioactive form of iodine is orally taken by the patient. As the reactive iodine is absorbed, the low level radiation is enough to destroy the overactive thyroid cells causing the thyroid to shrink and produce less hormones. The treatment is taken over several weeks. Patients may become hypothyroid more commonly if they have positive thyroid antibodies. A small number of people may develop Graves' disease from radioactive iodine.

Percutaneous Ethanol Injections (PEI)

This treatment or radiofrequency ablation may be used when surgery and radioactive iodine cannot be done. It involves injecting ethanol, an alcohol solution, into the nodule. This therapy requires a series of injections. This treatment has been shown to be safe and effective, especially with nodules which contain fluid.

Radiofrequency Ablation (RFA)

In this procedure, a needle electrode is inserted into the nodule through the skin. An electrical current produced by radio waves is used to heat up a small area contained within the nodule. This results in the destruction (ablation) of the nodule.

OUTCOME (PROGNOSIS)

The vast majority of AFTN treatments are highly effective. Side effects may range from hypothyroidism to Graves' disease. Where no serious symptoms are observed, your physician may ask that you come in for frequent check-ups to observe the AFTN.

MULTINODULAR GOITER (MNG)

Multinodular goiter occurs when a number of nodules are present on a partially or entirely enlarged thyroid gland. Most goiters are small, and produce no or few symptoms. When symptoms are present they are usually related to the growth and function of the thyroid. There are two forms of this type of goiter, non-toxic and toxic MNG. People that have a *non-toxic multinodular goiter* do not have any signs or symptoms and have normal thyroid function. In *toxic nodular goiter*, the individual usually has symptoms. Heart and gastrointestinal symptoms of hyperthyroidism are usually the most common. A multinodular goiter is usually slow to evolve and most often occurs in the elderly. Multinodular goiters are prevalent particularly in areas of the world that are iodine deficient.

Individuals with multinodular goiter may become hyperthyroid. Less commonly they become hypothyroid. The hyperthyroidism may develop insidiously. Commonly there is a long time of subclinical (undetected) hyperthyroidism where the patient will have low TSH and normal free T4 and T3. The hyperthyroidism is due to the growth of the goiter and also an associated increase in the mass of autonomously hormone-producing cells. The hyperthyroidism may also be due to use of iodine supplements or iodine containing drugs, such as amiodarone or dye. Transition from non-toxic goiter to toxic goiter is part of the development of the disease. The timeframe between when the goiter is non-toxic and becomes toxic is unknown.

RISK FACTORS

The risk factors for multinodular goiter are not clearly understood, however there are a number circumstances that researchers believe can lead to this condition.

Genetics

Genetics seem to play a role in a person's predisposition to develop MNG. However, it may require one or more triggers, as listed below, to initiate this condition.

Age

Statistics indicate the MNG occurs most often in people over age 60.

Environmental Conditions

Potentially any number of heavy metals and pollutants may build up triggering MNG.

Gender

Females are at higher risk to develop MNG than males.

SIGNS AND SYMPTOMS

The majority of multinodular goiters are non-toxic, show no symptoms and are only discovered during a physical exam. However, toxic multinodular goiters may show the following signs and symptoms:

❑ Enlargement of the thyroid gland during pregnancy

❑ Gradual development of hyperthyroidism

❑ Horner's syndrome (rare)

❑ Iodine-induced thyrotoxicosis

❑ Obstruction of the superior vena cava (superior vena cava obstruction syndrome)

❑ Obstruction of the thoracic inlet by extending the arms over the head (Pemberton's sign)

❑ Occasional cough and difficulty swallowing

❑ Phrenic nerve palsy (rare)

❑ Recurrent nerve palsy (rare)

❑ Slowly growing nodular anterior neck mass

❑ Sudden pain or enlargement secondary to bleeding (hemorrhage)

❑ Upper airway obstruction, shortness of breath, and tracheal compression

CAUSES

Goiters can materialize when the thyroid gland produces either too much or too little thyroid hormone. In the case of a non-toxic multinodular goiter, the enlargement can come about with a normal production of the thyroid hormone.

Iodine Deficiency

Studies have shown that populations that regularly consume iodized salt have much fewer cases of MNG than those communities that do not.

Smoking

The organic chemical thiocynate is generated when you smoke, and it may cause a goiter.

Medications

Taking medicines that contain iodine, such as amiodarone, may also lead to the disorder. Do not discontinue taking any medication without consulting your physician.

Diet

A diet high in natural goitrogens—substances that suppress the function of the thyroid gland by interfering with iodine uptake—may result in a goiter. Such as:

- Broccoli
- Cauliflower
- Kale
- Brussels sprouts
- Mustard greens
- Radishes
- Peaches
- Soy-based foods
- Peanuts
- Spinach
- Strawberries

While many of these foods are healthy for you, like anything else, it is important not to eat too much of one single food. Moderation is the key to health!

DIAGNOSIS

There are a number of tests available to determine whether you have a multinodular goiter (MNG).

Physical Examination

Normally, a physician can see some of the more pronounced signs, such a lump in the neck, thyroid enlargement, or signs of respiratory distress which can indicate MNG.

Blood Tests

The blood test is the most common test, and plays an important role in diagnosing thyroid disease and treating thyroid conditions. A number of blood tests will be done in order to determine if you are suffering from MNG.

Imaging Tests

Laboratory tests are not always accurate in diagnosing a dysfunction in the thyroid. Sometimes more tests are ordered. Imaging tests are administered for a diagnosis of various thyroid disorders. These can include an ultrasound, CT scan, MRI, scintigraphy (used for diagnosis test in nuclear medicine), or a PET scan.

Fine Needle Aspiration (FNA)

If MNG is found, a fine-needle aspiration is taken. The skin above the node is numbed and a thin needle is inserted into the area to remove cells for review. These samples are then sent to a laboratory where a pathologist examines them under a microscope to determine the exact nature of the cells. The pathologist writes up a report on his findings and sends back the report to the ordering physician.

TREATMENTS

Treatment of a multinodular goiter depends on the symptoms. Nodular thyroid disease is common. Many of these goiters do not cause major symptoms and may not need to be treated after proven non-cancerous. Treatment should be considered in the following cases:

- Cosmetic complaints
- Large goiter or progressive growth of entire gland or individual nodules
- Marked neck disfigurement
- Overt or subclinical hyperthyroidism
- Signs of cervical compression

There is no perfect treatment protocol for multinodular goiter. Treatments that are used include thionamides which are antithyroid medications, levothyroxine, surgery, or radioactive iodine.

Antithyroid Medication

Antithyroid medications, also called Thionamides, are used if a nodular goiter is complicated by hyperthyroidism. These drugs stop the production of TSH. Remission is rare, and usually treatment is indicated for life. Further growth may occur. Thionamides are also indicated before surgery to lower operative risk. To decrease the risk of making the hyperthyroidism worse, thionamides are suggested before radioactive iodine treatment.

Thyroid hormone therapy with levothyroxine for suppression of the pituitary TSH secretion has been used in the past, but since the natural progression of the goiter is to progress into hyperthyroidism, levothyroxine therapy is no longer suggested.

Surgery

The goal of surgery is to remove all thyroid tissue with a nodular appearance. Some surgeons remove part of the thyroid and other surgeons suggest the entire thyroid be taken out to prevent a recurrence. In the case of toxic nodular goiter, thyroid function is usually normalized more commonly with surgery than with radioactive iodine. Thionamides are not needed after surgery. Complications occasionally occur with surgery to the thyroid gland which may include infection, bleeding, vocal cord paralysis, and hypoparathyroidism. Rarely may other complications occur.

Radioactive Iodine (RAI)

Radioactive iodine is considered by many physicians as a safe treatment in many cases of hyperthyroidism, particularly in older people. It has a lower cost and less of a complication rate. Twenty to 40 percent of people will need a second dose of radioactive iodine. It causes the thyroid gland to shrink. It shrinks the same amount in toxic or non-toxic goiters. One possible complication of radioactive iodine treatment is radiation thyroiditis (inflammation of the thyroid gland) which is treated with steroids or salicylates. Another possible complication with radioactive iodine treatment is Graves' disease, an autoimmune type of hyperthyroidism, which is seen in about 5 percent of people.

If you have positive thyroid antibodies before treatment, the risk of Graves' disease is more common. This can also be seen after surgery and in subacute thyroiditis. Enlargement of the thyroid gland has not been seen after therapy. The risk of developing permanent hypothyroidism after radioactive iodine in multinodular goiters is from 14 percent to 58 percent within 5 to 8 years. This occurs more commonly in patients that have smaller goiter size to begin with and patients that have positive thyroid antibodies. The ability for radioactive iodine to work in multinodular goiter is decreased if there are a lot of nodules. Furthermore, a diet that is high in iodine makes treatment with radioactive iodine less reliable. Possible side effects of the treatment are hyperthyroidism and toxicity if larger doses are used.

Percutaneous Ethanol Injections (PEI)

This treatment may be used when surgery and radioactive iodine cannot be done. It involves injecting ethanol, an alcohol solution, into the nodule. This therapy requires a series of injections. This treatment has been shown to be safe and effective, especially with nodules which contain fluid.

PEI has been used for more than 10 years if there is only one node. More controlled studies need to be done. Possible risk factors include pain, risk of recurrent laryngeal nerve damage, and extrathyroidal fibrosis.

OUTCOMES (PROGNOSIS)

A multinodular goiter that causes no apparent symptoms is unlikely to cause problems over time, however it should be checked regularly by a physician. In the case of toxic multinodular goiters, immediate treatment should be undertaken. Because toxic multinodular goiters occur more commonly in people over 60, other chronic health issues, such as cardiovascular diseases and/or osteoporosis, may impact the outcome of the treatment.

SUBACUTE THYROIDITIS (SAT)

The term subacute thyroiditis refers to an inflammation of the thyroid gland. This is normally considered a self-limiting inflammatory disorder which means that it will run its course usually without treatment. It is the most common cause of pain, swelling, and discomfort in the neck area. It may be viral in origin.

Individuals with SAT may also experience symptoms of hyperthyroidism (see page 47) in its early stage and hypothyroidism (see page 24) in its late stage. In most patients, SAT lasts 2 to 4 months with some people having it for one year. About two-thirds of the people with SAT will have hypothyroidism as part of the disease process.

There are many names that subacute thyroiditis may be called, such as:

- Acute simple thyroiditis
- De Quervain's thyroiditis
- Diffuse or subacute thyroiditis
- Giant cell thyroiditis
- Granulomatous thyroiditis
- Migratory creeping thyroiditis

- Noninfectious thyroiditis
- Pseudo-giant cell thyroiditis
- Pseudogranulomatous thyroiditis
- Pseudotuberculous thyroiditis
- Viral thyroiditis

SIGNS AND SYMPTOMS

The patient may experience pain in one lobe, part of a lobe, or the whole thyroid. Pain may radiate from the thyroid gland to the angle of the jaw and to the ear of the affected side. If the pain is not bilateral at first, the pain and tenderness may spread to the other side of the thyroid within days or weeks. Pain may also radiate to the anterior chest or may be centered over the thyroid. When the patient moves their head, swallows or coughs it may aggravate symptoms. The following are possible early signs and symptoms of SAT:

- ❏ Evidence of thyroid dysfunction
- ❏ Fatigue
- ❏ Fever
- ❏ Pharyngitis (inflammation of the back of the throat)
- ❏ Weakness

Symptoms of mild-to-moderate hyperthyroidism may occur in the early phase in many people. Fifty percent of individuals have symptoms of thyrotoxicosis with nervousness, tremulousness, weight loss, heat intolerance, and tachycardia being the most common. Eight to 16 percent of people with SAT have a goiter before they developed SAT.

CAUSES

Subacute thyroiditis has also occurred in association with outbreaks of viral infections including the following:

- Adenovirus
- Cat-scratch fever
- Common cold
- Coxsackie virus
- Cytomegalovirus infection
- Hepatitis A
- Influenza

- Measles
- Mononucleosis
- Mumps
- Myocarditis
- Parvovirus B19 infection
- St. Louise encephalitis

SAT and SAT-like conditions have also occurred in association with other ailments, such as:

- Nonviral infections such as malaria and Q-fever
- Giant cell arteritis
- During interferon-alpha treatment for hepatitis C

- After long-term immuno-suppression and lithium therapy
- Following an allogeneic bone marrow transplant

Subacute thyroiditis is uncommon, but is more common in women who are 40 to 50 years old than in men. SAT more commonly occurs in North America, Japan, and Europe which are all temperate zones. Individuals may have positive thyroid antibodies that usually decrease or normalize as the SAT resolves. Some studies have shown a T-cell mediated immunity against thyroid antigens and/or a genetic link that may play a role in the pathogenesis of SAT. Complete recovery from subacute thyroiditis is common, but recurrence after several years has been reported.

DIAGNOSIS

If the patient has had a recent viral infection, based upon any of the infections described under causes (above), the physician may request any of the following tests to be run.

Blood Tests

Inflammatory blood markers, such as sedimentation rate (sed rate) and C-reactive protein, may be elevated. TSH is high, along with free T3 and free T4. Early on, liver enzymes may be elevated along with other blood studies. Thyroid antibodies may also be positive, in some cases a few weeks after the onset, and then decrease and disappear after the SAT is resolved. In a few individuals, SAT may trigger TSH receptor antibodies to be produced, which results in TSH antibody-associated dysfunction.

Imaging Tests

Imaging tests can be administered in considering the diagnosis of SAT. These can include an ultrasound, MRI, or color Doppler ultrasound test.

Urine Test

Urinary iodine levels may be high. Due to the increased urinary excretion of iodine, it may take more than one year for the iodine stores to be replenished.

TREATMENT

In some individuals no treatment is needed for SAT. Some will need aspirin or other anti-inflammatory medications or steroids if the case is severe. Recurrence rate is about 20 percent. Some people may develop hypothyroidism after they are treated.

Initially, some people will become hyperthyroid and many need to be treated with beta blockers. Sodium iopodate has also been used in the treatment of hyperthyroidism related to SAT. If you have numerous recurrences, then you are usually treated with thyroid medication if you are not hyperthyroid. This is to suppress TSH in order to reduce thyroid stimulation which prolongs the inflammation. Antibiotics have not shown to be effective.

If the case has gone on for many years, then removal of the thyroid gland may be suggested. Some people may become hypothyroid after treatment and then may require long term therapy with thyroid medication. Usually the hypothyroidism that may occur is transient, so that you lifelong thyroid medication is not needed.

OUTCOMES (PROGNOSIS)

In a majority of cases, subacute thyroiditis will need little medication, if any. However, if the condition continues for any length of time, the physician may prescribe any of the treatments related to hypo- or hyperthyroidism.

SILENT OR PAINLESS THYROIDITIS

Silent thyroiditis is an autoimmune process that presents with symptoms of thyroiditis (see page 47). Patients with this disease alternate between experiencing symptoms of hyperthyroidism and hypothyroidism. This condition is most commonly seen in women after delivery. It occurs in 5 to 9 percent of women in the first year after delivery particularly in women with positive thyroid antibodies. The course of the disease has four phases: thyrotoxicosis, euthyroidism (normal thyroid function), hypothyroidism, and euthyroidism. Not all four stages are present in all people. The usual course of disease is under 6 months for the toxic phase. The disease course is usually mild and generally you do not need treatment.

The incidence varies depending on where you may live. Silent thyroiditis is more common in Japan and uncommon in Argentina, Europe, and the east and west coasts of the United States. It is more common in the Great Lakes region and in Canada. Women up to the age of 60 and men may also be affected. Many people with silent or painless thyroiditis have a family history of the disease, including patients with postpartum thyroiditis. Exposure to iodine, such as in the form of amiodarone, lithium, interleukin-2, or interferon, may also be precipitating events. Painless or silent thyroiditis may be associated with other autoimmune diseases, such as rheumatoid arthritis, systemic sclerosis, Graves' disease, primary adrenal insufficiency, and lupus.

RISK FACTORS

The following are risk factors which may cause you to be more susceptible to this disease.

Child Birth

Due to the hormonal changes in the body of a pregnant and/or postpartum female, this condition may present itself.

Genetics

Genetics seem to play a role in a person's predisposition in developing this type of thyroiditis. If a mother developed this condition after giving birth then her daughter may develop thyroiditis after delivering a baby. However, it may require one or more triggers, as listed below, to initiate this condition.

Gender

Females are at higher risk to develop silent thyroiditis than males.

SIGNS AND SYMPTOMS

Symptoms are the same ones that you can see in thyrotoxicosis. (See page 47 for details.)

DIAGNOSIS

If the patient is postpartum, has an autoimmune disease, or has been exposed to iodine or medications that contain iodine, the physician my request any of the following tests to be run.

Blood Tests

Inflammatory blood markers, such as sedimentation rate (SED rate) and C-reactive protein, may be elevated. TSH, Free T3, Free T4, reverse T3, and thyroid antibody levels will determine the state of the thyroid gland.

Imaging Tests

Imaging tests can be administered to aid in the diagnosis of silent thyroiditis. These can include an ultrasound, MRI, or a color Doppler ultrasound test.

TREATMENT

The level of treatment is based on the severity of the condition.

Antithyroid Medications

Antithyroid medications prompt your thyroid gland to produce less thyroid hormone. These medications work faster than radioactive iodine therapy. Furthermore, you may take it before you have radioactive iodine therapy or surgery in order to restore your metabolism to normal.

Beta blockers (B-Adrenergic Antagonist Drugs). Beta blockers were originally designed to reduce blood pressure by blocking the effects of the adrenal hormone epinephrine, also called adrenaline. It does this by slowing down the heart's beats per minute as well opening up blocked vessels. This in turn reduces tachycardia, palpitations, tremor, and anxiety. The effects of B-adrenergic antagonists are fast, so it is important for use early on in the treatment of thyrotoxicosis. These drugs do not affect thyroid function, release, or synthesis.

Thionamides. They do not block the release of preformed thyroid hormone. Consequently it takes one to six weeks for the thyroid hormones that are already stored and the iodine that is stored to be depleted and for the patient to have total relief of symptoms and normalization of thyroid studies. Large goiters with large deposits of thyroid hormone may show a delayed response to thionamides. This drug may have a limited role.

Radioactive Iodine Therapy (RAI)

As discussed, in order to function, the thyroid gland needs to absorb iodine on a daily basis. With this therapy, a radioactive form of iodine is orally taken by the patient. As the reactive iodine is absorbed, the low level radiation is enough to destroy the overactive thyroid cells causing the thyroid to shrink and produce less hormones. The treatment is taken over several weeks. With the decrease in thyroid hormones the symptoms of Graves' is lessened.

Unfortunately, in cases where there is eye muscle irritation, the outcome is more complicated. For patients with mild inflammation of the eye muscles, the results may be mild and temporary, however in cases that are moderate to severe this therapy is not recommended. Nor is it recommended for women who are pregnant or nursing.

Because this treatment involves destroying thyroid cells, it will likely have an effect on the amount of thyroid hormones produced in the future. For that reason, a patient's thyroid hormone levels must be checked regularly, and that person may require thyroid medication to make up for a drop in thyroid hormone production.

Steroids

In more severe cases, such as subacute thyroiditis and thyroid storm, steroids are used short term.

OUTCOMES (PROGNOSIS)

In about half the cases, silent thyroiditis can go away on its own within one year. However for the remainder, their condition may develop into hypothyroidism immediately or present itself years later. The hypothyroidism can become permanent, in which case, they may be required to take a daily dose of thyroid hormone to keep their hormonal system in balance.

IODINE-INDUCED THYROTOXICOSIS (IIT)

Iodine-induced thyrotoxicosis (IIT), also known as Jod-Basedow phenomenon, is created when an increased or excessive amount of iodine enters an individual's system. In some, the IIT effect can occur with comparatively small increases in iodine intake based on preexisting thyroid dysfunctions. When this occurs it can lead to an iodine-induced hypothyroidism (see page 24) or thyrotoxicosis (see page 47). This condition may be temporary or it can become permanent.

There are also individuals who create their own self-Induced hyperthyroidism. This condition is known as factitious hyperthyroidism, and is more common than one would expect. For more information on this disorder, see inset on Patient-Induced Hyperthyroidism on page 99.

RISK FACTORS

The following are risk factors which may cause you to be more susceptible to this disease.

Genetics

Genetics is a risk factor for individuals who have a predisposition to thyroid diseases.

Individuals With Undetected Thyroid Disease

These individuals are people that have an underlying thyroid condition and are unaware of it.

Individuals Who Are/Or Have Been Treated for Either Hypo- Or Hyperthyroidism

In many instances, these patients have been prescribed iodine supplements or antithyroid drugs to keep their thyroid hormones in balance, and any additional iodine may cause IIT. For example, euthyroid patients previously treated with antithyroid drugs for Graves' disease and nontoxic diffuse or multinodular goiters with thyroid autonomy are prone to develop iodine-induced hyperthyroidism.

Geography

Individuals with thyroid conditions living in a region where iodine consumption is very low or high may be subject to IIT.

CAUSES

Normally, this condition arises due to an existing thyroid malfunction that is undetected or being treated. Iodine-induced thyrotoxicosis is caused by an excess amount of iodine entering the body. For some the excess amount of iodine may be minimal, while for others, it may require a much larger dose for the symptoms to appear.

Antithyroid Drugs

Drugs such as interferon alfa, lithium, and amiodarone are designed to disrupt the production of thyroid hormones, destroy thyroid cells, or do both. These drugs contain iodine concentrates which can lead to hypo- or hyperthyroidism. This can then make the individual susceptible to IIT.

Radioactive Iodine Dyes

When patients undergo scans requiring a radioactive iodine dye to observe the state of their thyroid gland, they may develop IIT.

Over-the-Counter and Prescription Drugs Containing Iodine

Drugs such as Iodochlorhydroxyquinoline, used in the treatment of prostate cancer, may bring on IIT due to its iodine content. Always ask you physician or pharmacist about the content of any other drugs you may be taking.

Antiseptics and Disinfectants

Many of the antiseptics and disinfectants used in hospitals and healthcare locations contain iodine. Tincture of iodine is commonly used on cuts and abrasions to kill bacteria.

Diet

A number of foods, such as shellfish, dried seaweed, cod, iodized salt, and to a lesser degree sea salt, contain iodine which have been shown to trigger IIT.

SIGNS AND SYMPTOMS

The onset of IIT may bring on many of the common issues associated with hypothyroidism and thyrotoxicosis. (See page 24 and 47 for details.)

DIAGNOSIS

There are a number of tests available to determine whether you have Iodine-induced thyrotoxicosis.

Physical Examination

An initial clinical diagnosis can be made based upon the medical history of the patient in conjunction with the identification of any of the possible causes of IIT listed above. When a diagnosis of IIT may be suspected, tests requiring the consumption of any substance containing iodine should be avoided. In addition, a standard examination to check blood pressure, body temperature, and heart rate will be made to determine the level of thyroid involvement.

Blood Tests

Inflammatory blood markers, such as sedimentation rate (sed rate) and C-reactive protein, may be elevated. TSH, Free T3 and Free T4, reverse T3, and thyroid antibody levels will determine the state of the thyroid gland.

TREATMENT

The treatment will depend on the cause and severity of the symptoms. It may require eliminating the underlying cause or drug therapy or both.

Eliminating Underlying Causes

When a cause can be identified, such as a specific food or antiseptic, avoiding the cause may reduce or eliminate the symptoms. When the cause is a medication, speak to your physician regarding its discontinued use. In some cases, there may be a severe or life-threatening reaction.

Drug Therapy

Based on the nature of the thyroid condition associated with IIT, thyroid replacement hormone is commonly prescribed if hypothyroidism is present. If the IIT has been brought about by the patient's use of amiodarone, and the thyroid is overactive, the IIT is treated with methimazole and potassium perchlorate when identified as Type I or with prednisone when identified as Type II.

OUTCOME (PROGNOSIS)

When treated early, iodine-induced thyrotoxicosis is usually transient, and normal thyroid function should return within two to three weeks. Because IIT involves regaining an appropriate amount of iodine in the body in relationship to the amount of thyroid hormones in the body, it is important to make sure that you have regular check-ups until the condition has been controlled or eliminated. Without an appropriate amount of thyroid hormones in the body, a number of serious life-threatening issues can occur.

Patient-Induced Hyperthyroidism

Although most cases of higher-than-normal thyroid hormone levels are caused by an overactive thyroid, this isn't always true. Sometimes, the problem occurs because the patient is taking too much thyroid hormone medication. This condition is known as factitious hyperthyroidism.

Patients take higher-than-prescribed doses of thyroid hormone for different reasons. In some cases, they use extra medication to lose weight, to control a menstrual disorder, to treat depression, or to treat infertility. In other cases, they have a psychiatric disorder such as Munchausen Syndrome—a mental illness in which the person wants to be seen as having a disorder even though she has caused the symptoms herself.

The diagnosis of factitious hyperthyroidism should be considered when laboratory tests and the physician's observations are contradictory. For instance, the individual's lab tests may reveal high levels of thyroid hormone, but they do not show the classic symptoms of Graves' disease (the most common form of hyperthyroidism), such as bulging eyes and goiter.

Symptoms of factitious hyperthyroidism normally disappear once thyroid medication dosage is lowered to the appropriate amount. If a psychiatric condition is responsible for the patient's excessive self-dosing, the individual will need mental health treatment to resolve the problem. Regardless of the cause, when factitious hyperthyroidism continues for a long time, it can take a heavy toll on the body. The patient should therefore be checked every two to four weeks to make sure that the thyroid levels have returned to a safe range.

ACUTE INFECTIOUS THYROIDITIS

Because iodine is a natural antiseptic, and it is stored in high amounts in the thyroid gland, it is normally resistant to infection. However, due to several existing conditions it can be infected by bacteria, mycobacteria, fungi, protozoa, or flatworms. When such an infection occurs this condition is called acute infectious thyroiditis. It can also be referred to as chronic infectious thyroiditis, suppurative (AST), nonsuppurative, or septic thyroiditis. These types of infections are normally rare.

RISK FACTORS

The following are risk factors which may make you more susceptible to this disease.

Abnormalities Of The Piriform Sinus

This is a condition where the lower sinus cavity (called the piriform sinus) or the space connecting sinus cavities (called a fistula) becomes infected and spreads the infection to the lower portion of the neck involving the thyroid.

Low Immune Condition

Individuals with lowered immunity function may be unable to fight off a variety of infections. Any infection, such as strep or strep bacteria, gaining a foothold in the neck area can lead to an abscess in the thyroid.

SIGNS AND SYMPTOMS

The following are symptoms you may experience when suffering from acute infectious thyroiditis:

❑ Fever and chills

❑ Local pain and tenderness in the affected lobe of the thyroid or the entire gland

❑ Painful swallowing and difficulty swallowing

❑ Pain may refer to the pharynx or ear and may be so prominent that the individual does not realize they have tenderness over their thyroid gland

DIAGNOSIS

If your physician suspects that you may have acute infectious thyroiditis a number of steps will be taken.

Physical Examination

A standard examination to check blood pressure, body temperature, and heart rate will be made to determine the level of thyroid involvement if any.

Blood Tests

Inflammatory blood markers, such as sedimentation rate (SED rate) and C-reactive protein, may be elevated. TSH, Free T3 and Free T4, reverse T3, and thyroid antibody levels will determine the state of the thyroid gland. A complete blood count may be done to look for infection along with other specialized studies.

Fine Needle Aspiration (FNA)

A fine-needle aspiration is taken. The skin above the node is numbed, and a thin needle is inserted into the area to remove cells for review. These samples are then sent to a laboratory where a pathologist examines them under a microscope to determine the exact source of the infection. The pathologist writes up a report on his findings and sends back the report to the ordering doctor.

TREATMENT

Based on the type of infection found, treatments usually include antibiotics or antifungal agents and may even include drainage.

OUTCOME (PROGNOSIS)

With the appropriate treatment, this condition is usually resolved.

HYPERTHYROIDISM AND PREGNANCY (GESTATIONAL TRANSIENT THYROTOXICOSIS)

Human chorionic gonadotropin (hCG) is a hormone that is produced in a pregnant woman. It has intrinsic TSH-like activity. In part, hCG is responsible for nausea during the first trimester of pregnancy. In 10 to 20 percent of normal pregnancies the hCG-induced hyperthyroidism goes undetected (subclinical). With multiple births, the hCG levels are even higher.

During the early stages of pregnancy, approximately 5 percent of woman experience nausea and vomiting along with weight loss. This is called hyperemesis gravidarum syndrome and is due to a woman's higher levels of hCG. Additionally, gestational transient thyrotoxicosis can also occur due to a gene mutation which makes the body hypersensitive to hCG.

Thyrotoxicosis can also be induced by a molar pregnancy and by tro-phoblastic disease. In a molar pregnancy with hyperthyroidism, studies have shown that when the hydatidiform mole is removed, the condition resolves.

RISK FACTORS

The following are risk factors which may make you more susceptible to this disease.

Pregnancy

Pregnancy brings on a number of hormonal changes in a woman's body. There is a rapidly rise in levels of estrogen and progesterone as well as hCG.

Genetics

Genetics is a risk factor for pregnant women who have a predisposition to thyroid diseases.

Preexisting Thyroid Disease

There may be a number of thyroid problems such as Grave's disease, an autoimmune-based disorder of the thyroid, which may have gone unde-tected prior to the pregnancy.

SIGNS AND SYMPTOMS

While some hGC-related symptoms are common during pregnancy, should these symptoms become excessive, you should contact your physi-cian and consider the possibility of checking your thyroid hormone lev-els. For a complete list of hyperthyroid symptoms see page 47.

❏ Diarrhea

❏ Enlarged thyroid gland

❏ Excessive sweating

❏ Fast heart beat (tachycardia)

❏ Mood changes

❏ Nausea

❏ Trouble sleeping

❏ Vomiting

❏ Weigh loss or gaining weight too slowly

DIAGNOSIS

If your physician suspects that you may have developed hyperthyroidism a number of steps will be taken.

Physical Examination

A standard examination to check blood pressure, body temperature, and heart rate will be made to determine the level of thyroid involvement if any.

Blood Tests

Results are normally based on high levels of T3 and Free T4 levels and low levels of TSH to determine the potential of hyperthyroidism.

Urine Test

Analyzing the thyroid hormone levels in the urine may be used as an adjunct to a blood test to indicate the status of the thyroid gland.

TREATMENT

With moderate hGC levels, there are usually no treatments necessary. Normally, this type of condition is termed "self-limited," since it will resolve itself after childbirth. When the symptoms are more severe, treatment is important, but may be limited owing to the safety of the baby. Treatments may include the following:

Anti-thyroid drugs. Of the three thionamide drugs, propylthiouracil (PTU) is preferred during first trimester of pregnancy. This drug is used to stop the production of TSH with fewer side effects.

Beta-blockers. These medications will be used to slow the mother's heart rate down and reduce tremors.

OUTCOME (PROGNOSIS)

For the majority of pregnant women, "morning sickness" is part of the ritual of having a baby. Its underlying cause is of little concern, since it clears up by the later stages of pregnancy. However, for some women, the symptoms may be much more severe and should be treated or at the very least, monitored by a physician. If left untreated, hyperthyroidism can have serious consequences to both mother and child.

CONCLUSION

While the majority of the thyroid-related disorders discussed in this chapter are relatively rare, to an individual who suffers from one of these conditions being rare means very little. What is important is identifying the problem, understanding what it is, and then knowing what your options are. Don't be afraid to ask your physician questions and act as your own advocate. As you will see in the upcoming chapters, your thyroid gland has a great deal to do with many aspects of your well-being.

6

Thyroid Hormones and Your Memory

hile you have seen how important thyroid hormones are to our overall metabolism, what you may not be aware of is the important role they play in keeping our brain functioning properly. As the center of our thought process, nervous system, and sensory capabilities, any chemical imbalances in this complex organ can have a significant impact in your daily lives. As you will see, such an impact can stem directly from improper thyroid hormone production—specifically on your ability to remember and focus.

Since thyroid hormones regulate every cell and organ of the body, it is not surprising that optimal thyroid hormone function is essential to the brain and its many activities, including the ability to form and preserve memory. Studies have shown that problems with the thyroid—even at a subclinical (undetected) level, when no obvious symptoms are present—can affect the brain in many ways.

This chapter first explores how thyroid hormone imbalances are known to influence a range of mental (cognitive) processes, including the acquisition of information, the ability to focus, the capacity to solve problems, and, of course, memory. It then looks at several specific forms of thyroid dysfunction, how they impact the brain, and how they can be treated.

AN OVERVIEW OF THE EFFECT OF THYROID PROBLEMS ON COGNITIVE FUNCTION AND MEMORY

Studies in both animals and humans have provided abundant evidence that thyroid hormone problems, whether they involve the production of too little thyroid hormone or too much thyroid hormone, can affect brain function in a number of ways. They can impair the growth of the neurons that allow the transmission of brain messages and they can influence the chemical substances vital to the transmission of these messages. Likewise, thyroid hormones affect other hormones, such as estrogen, progesterone, testosterone, DHEA, cortisol, and insulin, that also have a direct effect on memory, and they can furthermore directly affect the portion of the brain that's responsible for memory.

Hypothyroidism—an insufficient production of thyroid hormones (see Chapter 2)—has been found to impair neurogenesis, the growth and development of the neurons. Since neurons are the specialized cells that carry messages within the human brain, problems with neurogenesis can lead to reduced cognitive function. Normally, the thyroid hormones that are active in the brain have receptors that aid in carrying out these crucial activities. The thyroid hormone T3 has two receptors: alpha and beta which are paramount for focus and memory. Therefore, having enough levels of T3 is important.

The portion of the brain called the hippocampus is involved in forming, storing, and processing memory. As you might suspect, any condition that adversely affects this important structure also harms cognitive abilities. There are two hippocampus regions; one located on the left side of the brain, and the other on the right. These areas play an important role in storing short-term and long-term memory as well as giving you a sense of spatial navigation. In Alzheimer's disease, the hippocampus is one of the first areas of the brain to suffer damage resulting in memory loss or disorientation. When adult-onset hypothyroidism hampers hippocampal neurogenesis—the development of neurons within the hippocampus— both learning and memory are affected. Studies on animals have suggested that this impairment in memory may be related to damage to long-term potentiation (LTP), which is the strengthening of connections between neurons that supports signal transmission and enables the formation of memories. Fortunately, it has been found that replacement of T4—thyroxine, one of the thyroid hormones—can restore LTP and thus improve both learning and memory.

A number of studies have highlighted the importance of T4 to cognitive function. One study showed that when laboratory animals received T4 replacement, their learning ability for spatial tasks was enhanced. It is believed that the animals' improved learning was related to a healthier cholinergic system—the system that helps govern the learning process.

Studies have also demonstrated that levels of thyroid-stimulating hormone (TSH), which regulates the production of both T4 and T3 (triiodothyronine), are related to measures of attention, and that low levels of TSH may predict vascular dementia, a form of dementia caused by impaired blood supply to the brain.

T4 is not the only thyroid hormone that is involved in cognitive function. Both low *and* high levels of T3 have been found to result in severe cognitive problems. For instance, Graves' hyperthyroid patients—who have increased levels of T3—tend to experience problems with memory, attention, and complex problem solving. (See page 111 of this chapter for more about Graves' disease and cognition.) Optimal levels of T3 are vital for focus and memory.

Thyroid function has also been found to affect the function of neurotransmitters, the chemicals that transmit signals from one neuron to another neuron; as well as the function of neuromodulators, the chemicals that stimulate neuron function. As research continues, more will be learned about the many ways in which thyroid hormones influence memory and other cognitive abilities. At this point, studies have shown that optimal levels of thyroid hormones are vital for normal brain function.

FORMS OF THYROID DYSFUNCTION THAT AFFECT BRAIN FUNCTION

There are four common types of thyroid dysfunction that can affect cognition: overt hypothyroidism, subclinical hypothyroidism, overt hyperthyroidism, and subclinical hyperthyroidism. The remainder of this chapter examines these disorders and their relationship to focus and memory. Finally, this chapter looks at a rare form of thyroid dysfunction called Hashimoto's encephalopathy, which can have a profound effect on cognitive function.

OVERT HYPOTHYROIDISM

Overt hypothyroidism is hypothyroidism (low thyroid function) that can be measured by laboratory tests and manifests itself in obvious symptoms. It occurs when the thyroid gland is underactive and does not produce enough thyroid hormones.

Lab Findings

Tests of individuals with overt thyroid dysfunction show an increase in TSH, low levels of the hormone T4, and/or low levels of the hormone T3. (See Chapter 2 for more about hypothyroidism.)

Effects

In overt hypothyroidism, there is a widespread mild to moderate decrease in cognitive ability. Hypothyroidis.ι can decrease a number of brain functions, including general intelligence, general memory, the ability to pay attention and concentrate, perceptual function, language ability, psychomotor function (the relationship between brain function and physical movement), executive function (the mental skills that enable the brain to organize and act on information), and verbal memory (the memory of words and other aspects of language).

Test Results

Imaging studies performed on individuals with overt hypothyroidism have provided a good deal of physical evidence that brain function is altered in patients with this condition. Signs of overt hypothyroidism have been shown to include decreased blood flow; decreased function globally (throughout the brain), including areas that are necessary to attention and focus; decreased perception of the spatial relationships between objects in the individual's field of vision; decreased working memory—the system used to store and manage the information needed to learn, reason, and comprehend; and decreased motor speed—the speed at which body movement takes place.

Treatment

Fortunately, studies have shown that the replacement of T4 is helpful in most patients. For instance, in functional MRI (imaging) studies, hypothyroid individuals with decreased working memory experienced an improvement in memory after being treated with levothyroxine—a synthetic form of the T4 hormone—for 6 months. More studies need to be conducted, as additional patients might have improved if they had been treated with both T4 and T3.

If you are experiencing memory problems or other problems with cognitive function, it is worthwhile to consider the possibility that overt hypothyroidism is the root cause. To learn more about hypothyroidism, turn to Chapter 2, which will fill you in on the disorder's symptoms, methods of diagnosis, and possible forms of treatment, including not just thyroid replacement therapy but also detoxification, supplements, exercise, and diet.

SUBCLINICAL HYPOTHYROIDISM

Subclinical hypothyroidism is a mild form of hypothyroidism (low thyroid function) in which there are no obvious symptoms of thyroid trouble.

Lab Findings

Laboratory tests reveal only one abnormal hormone level: an increase in TSH or a TSH that is the upper limit of normal. Levels of T3 and T4 are usually within normal ranges. There is strong evidence that subclinical hypothyroidism is associated with a progression to an overt form of the disorder.

Effects

Smaller studies designed to evaluate patients for subtle cognitive impairment have shown that patients with subclinical hypothyroidism may display mild cognitive changes. The most commonly affected areas were memory and executive function. In one study, patients with subclinical hypothyroidism were shown to have impaired working memory, which means that they had trouble storing and using the information needed to learn, reason, and comprehend.

Test Results and Treatments

Functional MRI (imaging) studies have shown abnormal function in the frontal brain areas that are responsible for decision-making and planning. Some of the patients were treated with levothyroxine, a synthetic form of T4. This therapy resulted in normal working memory and normal function visible on the MRI.

PET scan imaging has revealed that individuals with subclinical hypothyroidism have lower-than-average glucose metabolism in the areas of the brain responsible for cognition. Since glucose is the brain's primary form of fuel, this indicates that subclinical hypothyroidism may compromise brain function, which is dependent on glucose. After 3 months of thyroid replacement therapy with T4, normal metabolic function was restored, enabling the brain to receive the energy it needs.

Although hormone therapy has been shown to help relieve cognitive problems associated with subclinical hypothyroidism, the treatment of this health condition is controversial, particularly when patients do not have recognized symptoms of thyroid disease, such as fatigue, increased

Subclinical Thyroid Conditions— To Treat or Not to Treat

While most physicians agree that thyroid levels which are clearly in "abnormal" ranges require treatment, the idea of treating subclinical hypothyroidism (see page 109) or subclinical hyperthyroidism (see page 112) is more controversial. Subclinical thyroid dysfunction is defined as a condition in which there is an abnormal TSH level—it is too high in hypothyroidism, and too low in hyperthyroidism—but the levels of the T3 and T4 thyroid hormones are within normal ranges. Doctors are especially reluctant to treat these disorders when the patient is not experiencing symptoms that are generally associated with thyroid dysfunction. But some physicians who work with patients who have psychiatric problems have demonstrated that the treatment of subclinical thyroid conditions can make an important difference, especially in the case of hypothyroidism.

In a study published in 2006, researchers in China provided patients who had subclinical hypothyroidism with levothyroxine therapy. Brain scans used before and after treatment showed significant improvements in both memory and executive function. Confirming these findings are anecdotal reports of psychiatrists who have had good results in treating people whose symptoms were often debilitating—even though their hypothyroidism was considered relatively minor. In fact, results of thyroid hormone therapy have been so encouraging that a few years after the study in China, researchers at Boston University began a trial to explore the connection between subclinical hypothyroidism and certain mood and cognitive disorders.

Although the results of the Boston University study are not yet known, many physicians believe that when an individual with subclinical thyroid problems is experiencing psychiatric or cognitive dysfunction, a trial of thyroid medication is warranted and—in the case of hypothyroidism—may even prevent future cognitive decline.

sensitivity to cold, and elevated cholesterol levels. (See the inset on page 110 for more about the treatment of subclinical thyroid problems.) Nevertheless, if you are experiencing cognitive problems, you should consider the possibility that they may be related to a subclinical form of low thyroid function. To learn more, turn to Chapter 2, which will fill you in on methods of diagnosis and possible forms of treatment, including not just thyroid replacement therapy but also detoxification, supplements, and diet.

OVERT HYPERTHYROIDISM

Overt hyperthyroidism is hyperthyroidism (higher-than-normal thyroid function) that can be measured by laboratory tests and manifests itself in obvious thyroid symptoms. It occurs when the thyroid gland is overactive and produces too much thyroid hormone.

Lab Findings

Tests of individuals with overt hyperthyroidism usually show a decrease in TSH and an increase in both T3 and T4 levels, although occasionally, the level of only one of these hormones is higher than normal. (See Chapter 3 for more about hyperthyroidism.)

Effects

Although memory and other cognitive problems seem to be more prevalent among people with hypothyroidism, a number of studies have shown an association between hyperthyroidism and cognitive disorders. People with Graves' disease, the most common cause of hyperthyroidism, are the most likely among hyperthyroid patients to report memory and concentration problems, as well as mood changes. Studies have shown that these symptoms can appear as much as two years earlier than other signs of the disorder. In fact, cognitive problems such as decreased memory and mood changes such as anxiety are often what lead patients to treatment in the first place.

Test Results

The subjective experiences of Graves' patients have been supported by functional imaging studies (PET scans), which have shown cerebral dysfunction, including abnormal glucose metabolism in the right hemispheric limbic system, which is a major region for long-term memory. (To learn more about Graves' disease, see Chapter 4.)

Treatment

In most studies, treatments designed to restore optimal thyroid function have resulted in improved cognition and emotional well-being in people with overt hyperthyroidism. In some studies, however, some residual attention deficits have remained even after the thyroid hormones were being produced in normal amounts.

If you are experiencing memory problems, attention problems, or mood changes, recognize that they may be caused by hyperthyroidism. To learn more about this condition, turn to Chapter 3, which will fill you in on the disorder's symptoms, methods of diagnosis, and possible forms of treatment, including medication, surgery, radioactive therapy, nutritional supplements, and diet. Be aware, though, that if you have Graves' disease and your symptoms include emotional changes such as nervousness, restlessness, and anxiety, your physician may conclude that you have a psychiatric problem such as generalized anxiety disorder. Too often, patients with Graves' are misdiagnosed because of these symptoms, causing delays in a true diagnosis and appropriate treatment. Make sure that your doctor performs the laboratory tests necessary to fully assess the reason for your condition.

SUBCLINICAL HYPERTHYROIDISM

Subclinical hyperthyroidism is a mild form of hyperthyroidism (higher-than-normal thyroid function) in which there are no obvious symptoms. Early Graves' disease, discussed above, accounts for the majority of subclinical hyperthyroidism cases. It has been found that few people with subclinical hyperthyroidism progress to an overt form of the disease.

Lab Findings

Laboratory tests reveal only one abnormal level: a decrease in TSH. Levels of T3 and T4 are within normal ranges.

Effects

The possible relationship between subclinical hyperthyroidism and cognitive problems is a controversial subject. Some studies show a connection, and some do not. Major cognitive problems are not usually seen, but mild problems with memory and concentration may be present. There is some evidence, too, that subclinical hyperthyroidism may be associated with an increased risk of developing dementia, but again, the findings have been conflicting. Subclinical hyperthyroidism appears to be more common in the elderly than it is in younger people.

Treatment

As explained earlier in the chapter, the treatment of subclinical thyroid problems is a subject of debate among doctors, especially when the individual doesn't have recognized symptoms of the disorder. (See the inset on page 110.) Nevertheless, if you are experiencing cognitive problems, a possible thyroid dysfunction should be investigated. Be aware, too, that subclinical hyperthyroidism can indicate the over use of thyroid hormones. In fact, this disorder is present in about 20 to 40 percent of subjects prescribed thyroid hormones, and may indicate overtreatment. So if you are on thyroid replacement therapy for *hypo*thyroidism and are experiencing cognitive or mood problems, it is a good idea to contact your doctor about the possible need to adjust your medication dose.

HASHIMOTO'S ENCEPHALOPATHY

Hashimoto's thyroiditis (first discussed on page 36) is an autoimmune disease and the most common cause of hypothyroidism (an underactive thyroid). Hashimoto's encephalopathy is a rare disorder of unknown cause that is associated with Hashimoto's thyroiditis.

Lab Findings

No specific diagnostic tests are available to detect Hashimoto's encephalopathy. The presence of some autoantibodies have been reported. In about 75 percent of reported cases, samples of the cerebrospinal fluid reveals an elevated level of proteins, but in 25 percent of the cases, this indicator is not present.

Effects

The symptoms of Hashimoto's encephalopathy are primarily neurological. Among them are memory and concentration problems as well as disorientation, seizures, tremor, myoclonus (rapid contraction and relaxation of muscles), and ataxia (lack of muscle control during voluntary movements, such as walking or picking up objects).

Test Results

Electroencephalography (EEG)—a record of electrical activity of the brain—is usually abnormal. This disease is difficult to detect, and diagnosis is usually performed through a process of exclusion.

Treatment

The treatment for Hashimoto's encephalopathy is steroid therapy, and rapid improvement can usually be observed within one to three days. Although this disorder is thyroid-related, it does not respond to thyroid therapy.

CONCLUSION

Optimal thyroid function is required for perfect focus and memory. As you have seen in this chapter, if thyroid hormone function is too high or too low, the condition may cause a decrease in focus and cognitive decline. It's important to recognize, too, that thyroid function imbalances which are allowed to continue without treatment can result in more serious health disorders over time. In a long-term trial that was part of the Framingham Study, it was found that women having either high or low levels of TSH had an increased risk of developing Alzheimer's disease, a degenerative disease for which there is no cure. Consequently, whenever cognitive problems are experienced, thyroid function should be checked and, if a problem is found, appropriate treatment should be initiated. In most cases this results in improved memory, focus, and overall brain function.

7

Thyroid Dysfunction and Your Mood

As you learned in Chapter 6, thyroid problems can affect the brain, which, in turn, can have an adverse effect on mental functions, such as the ability to create and preserve memory. Chapter 6 also touched on the fact that by acting on brain function, thyroid dysfunction can have an impact on mood. This chapter shines a spotlight on the link between the thyroid and mood changes.

The relationship between thyroid function and mood has been recognized for many years. Generally, an overactive thyroid (hyperthyroidism) can lead to anxiety, as well as nervousness, restlessness, and irritability. An underactive thyroid (hypothyroidism) is more likely to lead to depression. The more severe the thyroid disorder, the more severe the mood changes are likely to be.

This chapter first looks at neurotransmitters, the chemical messengers that not only send messages within the brain, but also have a profound effect on our emotional well-being. This is important, as one of the ways in which the thyroid affects mood is through its action on neurotransmitters. The chapter then takes a closer look at both depression and anxiety.

NEUROTRANSMITTERS

The brain is composed of over 100 billion nerve cells called neurons. It is through the neurons that the brain passes on information (or signals) that allow you to recognize and react physically and emotionally to both your internal thoughts and external stimuli, such as heat and cold. Every time you respond to an event or a feeling, every time you feel happy or sad, it is because of this system of message transmission.

Since neurons do not touch each other physically, but are separated by gaps called synapses, the messages (which are electrochemical signals) cannot move directly from one neuron to another. Instead, chemical neurotransmitters bridge the gaps, passing on the information from cell to cell. This happens very quickly, with millions of neurons being affected in an instant.

The brain produces two basic types off neurotransmitters.

- **Excitatory neurotransmitters.** These neurotransmitters promote the transmission of information from one neuron to another and have a stimulating effect on the body. They include aspartic acid, epinephrine (also known as adrenaline), glutamate, histamine, norepinephrine, and PEA (phenylethylamine).

- **Inhibitory neurotransmitters.** These neurotransmitters decrease the ability to transmit messages and have a calming effect on the body. These chemicals include agamatine, GABA (gamma-aminobutyric acid), glycine, serotonin, and taurine.

- **Dopamine.** This is a unique neurotransmitter in that it is both inhibitory and excitatory.

Each of the substances just named regulates specific functions in the body. Table 7.1 on page 117 gives you a clearer idea of the amazingly varied tasks that these vital chemicals perform, as well as symptoms of neurotransmitter deficiency and the foods that can increase production of each of these important chemicals.

As the table shows, in addition to performing a myriad of other functions, several neurotransmitters regulate mood. Serotonin is known as the "happy" neurotransmitter. When serotonin levels decrease in the body, feelings of depression, anxiety, or agitation may occur. Dopamine is another neurotransmitter that provides feelings of pleasure and enjoyment. GABA, histamine, and PEA also help regulate mood. It's important to understand, though, that *all* of the neurotransmitters are required for emotional well-being, as they interact with each other and with other chemicals in the body to maintain both physical and mental health. When the body produces the correct amount of these chemicals and they are in balance, your mood is positive and you feel upbeat and calm. When neurotransmitter levels are too high or too low, you can become depressed or anxious.

TABLE 7.1. NEUROTRANSMITTER FUNCTION AND DEFICIENCY

Functions		Symptoms of Deficiency
AGMATINE		
Aids wound healing Enhances immune function Enhances metabolism of fats Helps build proteins Helps produce glucagon and insulin Increases circulation	Increases production of growth hormone Increases sperm count Inhibits accumulation of plaque in the arteries Needed for digestive health Reduces pain from poor circulation	Agmatine deficiency is rare because the amino acid used in its manufacture is found in many foods and also made in the body.

Foods That Can Increase Agmatine Levels in the Body: Avocados; Beans; Brewer's yeast; Corn; Dark chocolate; Eggs; Green vegetables such as asparagus, broccoli, peas, and spinach; Meat; Dairy products; Nuts; Oatmeal; Onions; Potatoes; Raisins; Seafood; Seeds; Soy; Whole grains

ASPARTIC ACID		
Aids energy production from carbohydrate metabolism Assists production of DNA and RNA	Enhances immune system function Helps protect the liver from drug toxicity Increases energy and endurance	Depression Fatigue Reduced stamina

Foods That Can Increase Aspartic Acid Levels in the Body: Meat, Poultry, Seafood

DOPAMINE		
Controls the body's movements Maintains good concentration, memory, and problem-solving Provides feeling of enjoyment and pleasure, reinforcing certain behaviors	Regulates flow of information to other parts of the brain Stabilizes brain activity	Depression Excessive sleeping Inability to experience pleasure Tendency to crave and eat junk food, especially sweets Tendency to form addictions

Foods That Can Increase Dopamine Levels in the Body: Almonds, Avocados, Bananas, Beans, Dairy products, Poultry (especially turkey), Pumpkin seeds, Seafood (especially salmon), Sesame seeds

Functions		Symptoms of Deficiency
EPINEPHRINE (ADRENALINE)		
Constricts arteries	Addison's disease	Fatigue
Opens airways in lungs	Allergies	Low blood pressure
Quickens heartbeat	Constipation	
Raises blood pressure	Decreased tolerance to cold	Low blood sugar
Regulates blood pressure		Muscle weakness
Regulates mental focus		Need for excessive sleep
Strengthens force of heart's contractions	Depression or apathy	
Triggers release of glucose from energy stores		Poor circulation

Foods That Can Increase Epinephrine Levels in the Body: Beans, Dairy products, Eggs, Meat, Poultry, Tofu, Seafood

GABA		
Acts as muscle relaxant	Promotes secretion of growth hormone	Anxiety
Calms the brain		Insomnia
Lowers blood pressure	Relieves stress	Rapid heartbeat
Prevents anxiety		Seizures
		Sensation that brain is racing out of control

Foods That Can Increase GABA Levels in the Body: Beans, Brewer's yeast, Dairy products, Eggs, Fish, Legumes, Meat, Nuts, Seafood, Seeds, Soy, Whole grains

GLUTAMATE		
Balances blood sugar	Maintains muscle health	Glutamate deficiency is rare because this substance is found in many foods and manufactured in the body.
Decreases food cravings	Neutralizes toxins	
Enhances pain control	Plays a part in sensory perception	
Enhances sensory perception	Promotes healing	
Fuels the immune system	Promotes healthy acid-alkaline balance	
Improves mental alertness		
Increases energy	Promotes weight loss	
Maintains digestive health	Supports memory	
	Supports motor skills	

Functions		Symptoms of Deficiency
GLUTAMATE (cont.)		

Foods That Can Increase Glutamate Levels in the Body: Beans, Brewer's yeast, Brown rice, Dairy products, Eggs, Fish, Meat, Nuts, Seafood, Seeds, Soy, Whole grains

Functions		Symptoms of Deficiency
GLYCINE		
Aids absorption of calcium	Helps maintain the nervous system	Glycine deficiency is rare because this substance is found in many foods and manufactured in the body.
Aids in production of ATP, which stores energy within the cells	Needed to make bile acids	
Calms aggression	Needed to make glutathione, the body's most abundant natural antioxidant	
Decreases sugar cravings		
Helps build hemoglobin, proteins, DNA, and RNA	Promotes healthy prostate gland function	
Helps detoxify heavy metals in the body		

Foods That Can Increase Glycine Levels in the Body: Beans, Dairy products, Meat, Seafood

HISTAMINE	
Plays role in development of organs	Depression
Regulates mood	Hallucination
Signals immune system to react to allergens, causing an inflammatory response	Paranoia

Foods That Can Increase Histamine Levels in the Body: Citrus fruits, such as oranges and grapefruit; Garlic; Leafy green vegetables, such as spinach; Onions

NOREPINEPHRINE		
Constricts arteries	Quickens heartbeat	Depression
Enhances attention and focus	Raises blood pressure	Droopy eyelids
Increases blood flow to the muscles and brain	Regulates mental focus	Fatigue
Opens airways in lungs	Triggers release of glucose from energy stores	

Foods That Can Increase Norepinephrine Levels in the Body: Beans, Eggs, Meat, Dairy products, Poultry, Seafood, Tofu

Functions		Symptoms of Deficiency	
PHENYLETHYLAMINE (PEA)			
Elevates mood	Increases energy	Agitation	Decreased sexual interest
Enhances concentration	Promotes mental alertness	Confusion	Depression
		Decreased alertness	Fatigue
			Memory problems

Foods That Can Increase Phenylethylamine Levels in the Body: Bananas, Dairy products, Dark chocolate, Eggs • Do not eat foods that increase PEA if you have PKU.

Functions		Symptoms of Deficiency	
SEROTONIN			
Calms anxiety	Regulates sexual behavior	Anxiety	Loss of concentration
Controls appetite and carbohydrate cravings	Regulates sleep cycles	Cravings for sugar	Poor impulse control
		Depression	
Regulates body temperature	Relieves depression	Fatigue	
		Insomnia	

Foods That Can Increase Serotonin Levels in the Body: Beef, Chickpeas, Dairy products, Dates, Eggs, Peanuts, Poultry, Seafood, Sunflower seeds

Functions		Symptoms of Deficiency	
TAURINE			
Aids glucose metabolism	Improves liver function	Anxiety	Impaired vision
	Improves lung function	Depression	Infertility
Aids wound healing	Lowers blood pressure	High blood pressure	Kidney dysfunction
Boosts immune function	Lowers cholesterol		
Enhances use of calcium	Prevents blood clots	Hyperactivity	Seizures
Important for brain and nervous system function	Promotes kidney function	Hypothyroidism (low thyroid function)	
	Protects against cell membrane damage		
Important for visual pathways	Stabilizes heart rhythms		
Improves insulin sensitivity	Strengthens the heart muscle		

Foods That Can Increase Taurine Levels in the Body: Brewer's yeast, Dairy products, Eggs, Fish, Meat, Seafood • Avoid foods that contain MSG, since MSG degrades taurine.

NEUROTRANSMITTERS AND THE THYROID

What is the relationship between neurotransmitters and the thyroid? A number of studies have shown that low levels of thyroid hormones lead to low levels of neurotransmitters, including those neurotransmitters that have been shown to influence mood. For instance, low thyroid hormones can cause a decreased production of the neurotransmitter dopamine, leading to depression and the loss of motivation and willpower. Insufficient production of thyroid hormones can also decrease the levels of GABA and serotonin—two other neurotransmitters vital to the regulation of mood.

Further studies are needed to explain the complex interaction between the thyroid, the neurotransmitter system, and your emotions. For the time being, if you think you are experiencing the symptoms of neurotransmitter dysfunction, the only way to know for sure is to see a physician that specializes in Metabolic, Functional, or Personalized Medicine. (See Resources.) This specialist can arrange for urine tests that can detect neurotransmitters and their metabolites. Try to improve your diet to include some of the healthy neurotransmitter-stimulating foods listed in Table 7.1 on page 117. Finally, consider the possibility that your thyroid hormone production may be low and affecting the levels of your mood-balancing neurotransmitters. Below, you'll learn more about the relationship between thyroid dysfunction, depression, and anxiety.

DEPRESSION

Depression is the most common mental health condition, reportedly affecting one in ten Americans at some point in their lives. In any given year, more than 19 million people in the United States are estimated to suffer from depression. In fact, this illness has been called the "common cold" of mental health disorders. Moreover, it is rapidly becoming a significant health concern worldwide.

What Is Depression?

Depression is a medical disorder that involves both the mind and the body. Far more than a case of the blues, it is a feeling of unhappiness, melancholy, or despair that lasts for a prolonged period of time—weeks, months, or even years. It often recurs over time, requiring long-term treatment, just like diabetes or heart disease.

Although depression is sometimes thought of as being extreme sadness, there is a big difference between sadness and clinical depression, which is also called major depression and major depressive disorder. Everyone experiences sadness at some time in their lives, usually as the result of unpleasant circumstances, such as the loss of a job or the death of a loved one. In time, the sadness lifts as the individual deals with life's problems. But in the case of clinical depression, the feelings last much longer and the individual often does not know their cause. Furthermore, while people who are sad usually manage to cope with life and perform everyday activities, those who are clinically depressed may feel overwhelmed and unable to deal with common tasks. Moreover, depression usually includes some symptoms—such as backache—that are not associated with a temporary case of the blues.

What are the Symptoms of Depression?

The symptoms of depression can vary from person to person, and also according to age. Below, you will find the signs and symptoms that are characteristic of adult depression. Following this, you will find symptoms of depression that are specific to certain age groups. Be aware that older adults may also have the common signs of adult depression, but that some of these problems—fatigue, loss of appetite, and reduced interest in sex, for example—typically go unrecognized because they are seen as being part of aging or another illness. It is important to recognize *all* behaviors and feelings to determine if you or someone you know is suffering from depression.

Common Symptoms of Adult Depression

- Agitation or restlessness, resulting in hand-wringing or pacing
- Crying spells without cause
- Decreased appetite and weight loss
- Increased appetite and weight gain
- Excessive sleeping
- Fatigue
- Feelings of sadness
- Feelings of worthlessness or guilt
- Frequent thoughts of death or suicide
- Frustration and irritability, even over small events
- Indecisiveness

- Insomnia
- Intense cravings for certain foods
- Loss of concentration
- Loss of interest in activities that are normally pleasurable

- Reduced sex drive
- Slowness in thinking, speaking, or moving
- Unexplained physical problems such as backache

Symptoms Characteristic of Adolescent and Teen Depression

- Anxiety and anger
- Avoidance of social situations
- Behavior and mental health problems such as attention deficit hyperactivity disorder (ADHD)

Symptoms Characteristic of Older Adult Depression

- Desire to stay home
- Feelings of boredom and dissatisfaction with life
- Thoughts of suicide

What Is the Treatment for Depression?

A combination of treatments may be used to relieve depression. Treatment may include various types of antidepressants and/or some form of psychotherapy, such as cognitive therapy, interpersonal therapy, behavioral therapy, or problem-solving therapy. Although a depressive disorder can be debilitating, hindering the individual's ability to work, sleep, and eat, only about half of Americans who have major depression receive help. Many people resist treatment because they believe that the condition isn't serious, that they can manage it themselves, or that the disorder is a sign of personal weakness. This is unfortunate, as about 70 percent of those who seek medical help experience significant improvement and depression is just like any other illness such as hypertension or diabetes. It has nothing to do with personal weakness.

Of course, to a large degree, successful treatment depends on understanding the cause of the depression. If the root cause is thyroid dysfunction, that problem must be resolved in order to restore emotional well-being.

Depression and Thyroid Dysfunction

Depression has long been known to be a common symptom of hypothyroidism, or low thyroid function. (See Chapter 2 for more about hypothyroidism.) In fact, subclinical (undetected) hypothyroidism—a relatively mild form of the disease, in which no obvious signs of thyroid problems are seen—has been found present in up to 40 percent of patients with depression. It is believed that hypothyroidism can lead to depression in a number of ways.

- As you learned earlier in the chapter, hypothyroidism can cause this condition by decreasing the production of neurotransmitters. Neurotransmitters such as serotonin, dopamine, and GABA are needed in optimal amounts to maintain emotional health. When thyroid function is abnormally low, it causes levels of these chemicals to drop, as well, and depression can result.

- Hypothyroidism can also influence mood by affecting the mitochondria, which are the cell structures that create energy. Thyroid hormones are essential for both the formation and the function of the mitochondria, so when thyroid function is insufficient, fatigue, depression, and foggy thinking can result.

- Thyroid dysfunction can also cause depression by affecting the balance of a myriad of hormones, including estrogen, progesterone, testosterone, and DHEA, pregnenolone, and cortisol. Hormone imbalance prevents the body from managing stress and experiencing positive moods.

According to the American Association of Clinical Endocrinologists, whenever a patient is diagnosed with a depressive disorder, subclinical or clinical hypothyroidism should be considered. In fact, the link between these two disorders is so well known that thyroid medications—such as liothyronine (synthetic T3 hormone) and levothyroxine (synthetic T4 hormone)—are sometimes added to antidepressant treatment even when thyroid function has been found normal in laboratory tests. The Sequenced Treatment Alternatives to Relieve Depression (STAR*D) study showed that the combination of T3 thyroid hormone and antidepressants resulted in additional improvements in about 25 percent of subjects whose major depression had not been relieved by antidepressant therapy alone. One theory is that thyroid drugs and antidepressants work synergistically to boost each other's effects. Another possibility is that thyroid pills stimulate chemical activity in the brain, enhancing both mood and concentration. Whatever the mechanism involved, it is clear that when depression is a problem, and especially when standard treatments provide little if any improvement, the possibility of thyroid dysfunction should be explored.

ANXIETY

Like depression, anxiety is a common mental health condition. In any given year, some form of anxiety affects about 18 percent of the US population. It is estimated that each year, 40 million Americans experience anxiety symptoms severe enough to disrupt their daily activities, including job performance, school work, and relationships.

What Is Anxiety?

Anxiety is a feeling of worry, nervousness, or unease. Although these are normal human emotions that often occur in times of difficulty, an anxiety disorder is a serious mental illness that persists for an extended period of time and interferes with the ability to lead a normal life. For some people, anxiety can be crippling.

It's important to understand that there are several different types of anxiety disorder. The four major forms include:

- **Generalized anxiety disorder (GAD).** Those who have generalized anxiety disorder often experience excessive worry and fear over situations that for most people are not threatening.

- **Panic disorder.** Individuals who have panic disorder experience feelings of terror that strike suddenly and repeatedly, usually without warning. Symptoms—which can include sweating, chest pain, irregular heartbeat, and more—can be so severe that the person may feel that they are having a heart attack.

- **Social anxiety disorder.** People with this form of anxiety, which is also called social phobia, experience overwhelming self-consciousness and worry about everyday social situations. Their worry is often based on an extreme fear of being judged harshly by the people around them.

- **Specific phobias.** Individuals with specific phobias have an intense fear of a particular object or situation, such as spiders, thunderstorms, or flying in an airplane. The level of fear is so great that the person often avoids common situations.

What Are the Symptoms of Anxiety?

The symptoms of anxiety can vary from person to person, and, of course, they also vary according to the type of anxiety disorder involved. The Anxiety and Depression Association of America (ADAA) lists the following as general symptoms of anxiety:

❏ Chest pain or discomfort

❏ Chills or heat flashes

❏ Difficulty breathing, such as shortness of breath or the sensation of smothering

❏ Fear of dying

❏ Feelings of dizziness, unsteadiness, or light-headedness

❏ Feelings of unreality or of being detached from oneself

❏ Nausea or abdominal distress

❏ Palpitations, including a pounding heart or accelerated heart rate

❏ Sweating

❏ The sensation of choking

❏ Trembling or shaking

What Is the Treatment for Anxiety?

Anxiety disorders are very treatable, and, like depression, a variety of treatments may be used. The most common methods of treatment are medications, including traditional anti-anxiety drugs, antidepressants, and beta-blockers; and psychotherapy, such as cognitive behavioral therapy. Alternative approaches, such as biofeedback and calming herbs, are also used.

Only about a third of people with anxiety disorders seek treatment. However, most cases of anxiety disorder—even severe cases—can be treated successfully, with most patients feeling substantial relief within a few months.

Anxiety and Thyroid Function

As you learned in Chapter 3, hyperthyroidism occurs when the thyroid gland overproduces thyroid hormone. Anxiety is considered one of the most common symptoms of an overactive thyroid.

How does hyperthyroidism cause anxiety? Because thyroid hormones activate the entire body, an overproduction of these hormones causes the nervous system to be more active, potentially causing nervous tremors and shaking, sleeplessness, a racing heart, and irritability—all of which are symptoms of anxiety. This is why it's often difficult to tell the difference between true anxiety and hyperthyroidism.

As explained earlier in the chapter, hyperthyroidism can also cause mood disorders by upsetting the balance of your neurotransmitters, the chemicals that send messages within the brain and also help regulate mood. The function of chemical neurotransmitters is intimately affected by your body's hormones, and when levels of thyroid hormones are too high, neurotransmitter production is disrupted, potentially causing anxiety.

Although we don't know all the ways hyperthyroidism is associated with anxiety, studies have found that an overproduction of thyroid hormones is the most frequent medical condition misdiagnosed as anxiety disorder. This means that in cases of anxiety, the possibility of an overactive thyroid should always be considered.

CONCLUSION

Because the thyroid gland affects every cell in the body, thyroid function has an influence on every body function. Small wonder, then, that when the thyroid malfunctions, your mood can suffer.

If you are experiencing depression or anxiety, it makes sense to request tests designed to detect thyroid problems. Remember that it is not uncommon for thyroid dysfunction to be misdiagnosed as a disorder with psychological rather than physical roots. Treatments that restore normal function of the thyroid gland, whether used alone or with other therapies, may be able to restore your emotional well-being.

8

Thyroid Hormones and Your Heart

There are many reasons why people experience health issues related to their heart—lack of exercise, eating the wrong foods, and a family history of heart troubles. However, it has been found that common signs and symptoms of thyroid disease may be a result of how thyroid hormones affect the heart and the cardiovascular system. If you have been diagnosed with hyperthyroidism (see Chapters 3 and 4 for details describing hyperthyroidism) and experiencing frequent palpitations or a high heart rate, these heart issues may be directly associated with this condition. Heart related disorders can be associated with an undiagnosed or untreated thyroid dysfunction with hypo or hyperthyroidism. As the evidence will show, thyroid hormone balance is necessary for optimal heart function!

The thyroid is the body regulator, and therefore it is crucial that the thyroid gland functions perfectly and not just normally to help prevent heart disease and treat cardiovascular disease. Thyroid disorders can directly affect the normal function of the heart resulting in serious symptoms and cardiac complications. Thyroid dysfunction as hypothyroidism or hyperthyroidism can both have a negative impact upon cardiovascular health and are risk factors for heart disease. Thyroid hormones, T4 and T3 (see page 7), are important managers of cardiac function and cardiovascular blood flow.

This chapter provides you with an overall look at the importance of thyroid hormones and a healthy thyroid gland for optimal function of your heart. Presented are the symptoms of a dysfunctional thyroid, how hypothyroidism and hyperthyroidism can affect the heart, and cardiovascular risk factors associated with a dysfunctional thyroid. In addition, this chapter will offer a number of important tests and effective treatments.

IMPORTANCE OF T4 AND T3

A healthy heart and cardiovascular system is highly dependent on sufficient levels of T3. This active hormone regulates your metabolism, clearing out excess arterial fatty deposits. T4 is largely considered by many researchers to be an inactive prohormone; that is, it is precursor to another hormone it will turn into. Most of the T4 produced by the body is converted to T3 (see page 7). T3 is then delivered to particular organs that use predominately T3, such as the heart. Severe illness that is chronic, such as heart disease, is commonly associated with low T3 levels in the blood. This is called "low T3 syndrome." Actions of T3 at the cellular level have significant affects upon the heart.

Studies have shown that it is T3 and not T4 which enters a white blood cell that then enters the blood and attacks bacteria and viruses (this cell is the cardiac monocyte). Furthermore, it is the calcium cycling proteins in the heart that are the most important target of the action of thyroid hormone. Other heart functions, such as the transport of calcium (ATPase), and the control of cardiac self-contraction (phospholamban), are regulated by T3. If there is not enough T3 present, then impaired diastolic function of the heart may occur. The heart muscles may not relax in a normal manner which will result in the heart filling with blood too slowly or too quickly.

T3 also has direct effects on the mitochondria, which are rod-shaped structures that create energy and assist in the cell's function. In addition, hearts that are low in T3 show poor absorption of glucose, lactate, and free fatty acids by the mitochondria that power the heart cells. On the other hand, higher blood levels of T3 have been shown to be associated with improved heart function by increasing contractility, improved diastolic function, and lower systemic vascular resistance. Heart rate is one of the most sensitive physiological measurements of optimal thyroid function, and as it turns out, heart rate is also associated with serum T3 levels.

As we can see, medical research has shown that thyroid hormones are crucial to the daily operation of the heart. Now let's look at the effect of hypothyroidism and hyperthyroidism on heart function.

HYPOTHYROIDISM AND THE HEART

Many scientific studies have shown that hypothyroidism is connected with an increased risk for cardiovascular disease, mainly heart disease.

The heart is a major destination for thyroid hormones and any significant change in thyroid hormones will cause the heart to react. An underactive thyroid, producing a decreased amount of thyroid hormone, generally results in your heart beating too slowly, your blood pressure changing, and a rise in the cholesterol level in your blood.

SIGNS AND SYMPTOMS

Individuals with low thyroid function (hypothyroidism) may have specific signs and symptoms that are related to the cardiovascular system.

❏ Decreased endothelial derived relaxation factor

❏ Decreased endurance

❏ Diastolic hypertension (high blood pressure)

❏ Elevated c-reactive protein (CRP)

❏ Fatigue

❏ Impaired cardiac contractility

❏ Impaired diastolic function

❏ Increased homocysteine (an amino acid)

❏ Increased serum cholesterol

❏ Increased systemic vascular resistance

❏ Mitral valve prolapse (more common in patients with Hashimoto's thyroiditis)

❏ Narrow pulse pressure

❏ Slow heart rate (bradycardia)

HYPOTHYROIDISM AND CARDIOVASCULAR COMPLICATIONS

There are a number of specific markers that can indicate the possibility of you developing heart issues. You have a greater chance of developing cardiovascular problems if you are suffering from more than one risk factor.

Atherosclerosis. People with hypothyroidism may have an increased risk of developing heart disease since they may have a higher rate of hardening of the arteries (atherosclerosis). Trials have also shown an increase in abdominal aortic atherosclerosis in patients with mild hypothyroidism.

Cardiac fibroblasts. Hypothyroidism may promote an abnormal thickening of the heart valves (myocardial fibrosis) by stimulating fibroblasts, which is the opposite of which occurs in hyperthyroidism. Cardiac fibroblasts are the largest cell group in the heart and they contribute to the structural, biochemical, mechanical, and electrical properties of the myocardium.

Cholesterol. One study showed a direct relationship between the level of TSH and serum total cholesterol and LDL (bad cholesterol). High cholesterol can be affected by your thyroid and it can alter your heart health. Furthermore, it can lead to strokes since plaque can build up in your arteries elsewhere in your body.

Creatine kinase. Trials have also shown that serum creatine kinase (enzyme found in the heart) is elevated by 50 percent in about 30 percent of patients with hypothyroidism. An elevated level of creatine kinase is seen within hours of a heart attack, when the heart muscle is damaged. Also, fluid around the heart (pericardial effusions) may occur due to the increase in volume of distribution of albumin and the decrease in lymphatic clearance that may occur commonly in patients with hypothyroidism.

Low T3 levels. Trials in both humans and animals have shown that low thyroid hormone levels contribute to a poorer outcome after acute myocardial infarction (heart attack). A rapid decline in free T3 was found during the first week after a heart attack. Reverse T3 also was increased, but free T4 remained normal. Another study showed that in-hospital and post-discharge death rate was higher among individuals with lower T3 levels and higher reverse T3 levels.

Statin drugs. Some people have difficulty taking statin drugs to lower their cholesterol since the medications in some individuals are associated with the development of a cardiac myopathy (a muscular disease). This myopathy has been associated with low coenzyme Q-10 levels. It has also been shown that the myopathy that can be caused by statin drugs may be associated with mild thyroid insufficiency. Consequently, all patients taking a statin drug should be evaluated for hypothyroidism and treated if appropriate.

DIAGNOSIS AND TREATMENT

The first step in determining if you may be suffering from heart disease is getting a doctor's exam. Your doctor will then decide which test to administer in order to make a diagnosis.

Echocardiogram

An Echocardiogram (ECHO) is an ultrasound that measures how electrical impulses move through heart muscle allowing your doctor to view your heart beating and pumping blood. The echocardiogram shows mild to moderate large pericardial effusions in up to 30 percent of people with severe hypothyroidism. The pericardial output however is usually not decreased. When the individual is prescribed thyroid hormone the fluid around the heart usually resolves in a few weeks to a few months.

Electrocardiogram

An Electrocardiogram (EKG) is a static picture of the heart used to assess your heart rhythm, to measure the heart flow to the heart, to diagnose an enlarged heart, and to diagnose a heart attack. The EKG changes in patients with hypothyroidism may include any of the following:

- Lengthened duration of contraction which predisposes people to ventricular arrhythmias (irregular heart rhythms)

- Low voltage

- Sinus bradycardia (slower than average heart rate)

SUBCLINICAL HYPOTHYROIDISM

Subclinical (undetected) hypothyroidism is categorized as a moderate form of hypothyroidism. It is an early phase of the disease and it has none or few clinical symptoms that are detectable. Individuals with subclinical hypothyroidism are usually people with elevated TSH levels but have normal serum free or total T4 and normal free T3. The incidence of subclinical hypothyroidism increases with age. In younger patients it is more common in women. In older people the rate is evenly split between men and women. Several studies have shown a strong link between subclinical hypothyroidism and poor outcome in people with and without heart disease. In patients with chronic heart failure, TSH levels that are even slightly above normal are found to be independently associated with an increased risk of progression of heart failure. This is one of the reasons that it is important to treat subclinical hypothyroidism.

There are changes that may occur in thyroid metabolism in patients with heart disease. Interestingly, an alteration may occur in the metabolism of thyroid hormone if the patient has heart disease, has had heart surgery, or has had a heart attack. Commonly you may have a low free T3 with normal TSH and free T4 levels. Furthermore in people with heart failure there is commonly a decrease in serum T3 concentration which is usually proportional to the severity of the disease.

Low T3

If the person has a low ratio of T3 to reverse T3, it is a predictor of mortality if the individual has congestive heart failure. Studies have shown that if the patient is given T3 then the cardiac output is increased and the systemic vascular resistance is decreased and the patient improves. An abnormal heart rhythm (ventricular tachycardia) has been shown to be associated with low T3 or low T3/T4 ratio and increased levels of reverse T3. In fact, one study showed that elevated reverse T3 levels were the strongest predictor of mortality in the first year after having a heart attack. Low T3 has also been shown to be predictive of developing abnormal heart rhythm (atrial fibrillation) after having open heart surgery. Furthermore, low T3 levels are a strong predictor of death in patients with heart disease. Another study showed that thyroid hormone dysfunction plays an important role in the progression to dilated cardiomyopathy which is a syndrome where the heart gets larger and eventually fails. When the subjects in the study were given thyroid hormone replacement, they had significant improvement.

Again, it is very important that the patient have optimal thyroid function in many aspects, but particularly when it comes to the prevention and treatment of heart disease. Women with TSH levels in the upper reference range have increased arterial stiffness compared to women with lower TSH. This increases their risk of heart disease. This study was done on postmenopausal women. T3 is also important in the regulation of cardiac gene expression. Furthermore, the list of T3-mediated genes that are changed in hypothyroidism are very similar to the changes in gene expression in heart failure.

Signs and Symptoms

If your physician believes that you may be suffering from subclinical hypothyroidism because you may be experiencing mild symptoms, such as fatigue, depression, consistent weight gain, or memory problems, he/she may order lab tests to support the diagnosis. If you are diagnosed with subclinical hypothyroidism, it should be monitored and treated to achieve optimal thyroid function and to decrease the risk of heart disease. Other signs and symptoms of subclinical hypothyroidism that are related to the cardiovascular system are:

- Cholesterol levels increase parallel with an increase in TSH levels about 5 mU/L

- Higher rate of hardening of the arteries, altered cardiac contractility, and systemic vascular resistance.

- Independent risk factor for atherosclerosis and heart attack in female patients

- Positive thyroid antibodies increases the risk of acute myocardial infarction

Treatment

Research has shown and recommended that, from a cardiac perspective, patients with subclinical hypothyroidism be treated with thyroid hormone. A medical trial, of patients with subclinical hypothyroidism, showed benefits on cardiovascular risk factors and quality of life when they were supplemented with thyroid hormone. Another study also showed that after thyroid hormone replacement lipid (cholesterol) levels improved, resistance to pumping blood (systemic vascular resistance) lowered, and the ability of heart self-contraction (heart contractility) was also improved.

One study showed that heart disease mortality in female patients and also abnormal serum lipids for people were more common if they had subclinical hypothyroidism. Lastly, a study done using the United Kingdom General Practitioner research database revealed an important finding. It found that 53 percent of people who were under the age of 70, that were treated with levothyroxine for their subclinical hypothyroidism, had a reduction in recurring chest pain or discomfort (ischemic heart disease events), as well as death from cardiovascular disease.

Low T3 syndrome has been found to be a strong prognostic, independent predictor of death in people with acute and chronic heart disease. Likewise, patients with heart disease that have normal thyroid function were found to have lower levels of T3 compared to healthy patients. Consequently, it is imperative that when evaluating thyroid function in people with subclinical hypothyroidism that optimal levels of thyroid hormone be achieved and that T3 also be replaced along with T4.

OTHER MARKERS FOR INCREASED RISK OF HEART DISEASE ASSOCIATED WITH HYPOTHYROIDISM

Thyroid gland disorders can directly change the normal role of the heart causing symptoms and resulting in serious complications. For example, additional key indicators for increased risk of heart disease are elevated levels of C-reactive protein (CRP) and homocysteine in the blood. These markers can also be linked to hypothyroidism. Improving an underactive thyroid condition can also improve your cardiovascular health.

C-reactive Protein (CRP)

C-reactive protein is a marker for inflammation in the body and is a major risk factor for cardiovascular disease. CRP is produced in the liver, and it is measured by administering a blood test. Elevated levels occur when there is inflammation in the lining of the arteries which leads to the formation of plaque and eventually a narrowing of the walls of the blood vessels.

Causes of Elevated Levels

Elevated levels of CRP are caused by infection and many long-term conditions, such as cancer, lupus, pain resulting from swelling of the blood vessels (giant cell arteritis), rheumatoid arthritis, infection of the bone (osteomyelitis), rheumatic fever, tuberculosis, and inflammatory bowel syndrome. Elevated levels of CRP are also seen in some patients at menopause and also in some women with polycystic ovarian syndrome (PCOS). High levels of CRP may furthermore be a risk factor for diabetes and hypertension. When evaluating the patient for heart disease, commonly your doctor will order a special kind of C-reactive protein test called high-sensitivity CRP (hs-CRP).

Test Results

The following are recommendations made by the American Heart Association in relation to cardiovascular risk and CRP levels:

- 1 mg per liter or lower is regarded as low risk

- 1 to 3 mg per liter is regarded as moderate risk

- 3 mg or greater is regarded as high risk

- levels higher than 10 mg per liter may indicate a heart attack or a great risk of having a myocardial infarction

Treatment

You can lower your CRP level with natural foods, diet, vitamins, omega-3 fatty acids, herbs, and supplements. Specifically, the following are ways to lower C-reactive protein:

- Antibiotics (if an infection is present or levels are very elevated)

- Baby aspirin, one per day (check with your doctor first)

- Balancing hormones in women with PCOS

- Coenzyme Q-10

- Curcumin (200 to 600 mg a day)

- Essential fatty acids such as fish oil or EPA/DHA (1,000 mg a day)

- Grapeseed extract (100 to 200 mg per day)

- Green tea (3 cups per day)

- Moderate exercise

- Natural estrogen replacement in menopausal women that are deficient and are able to take estrogen

- Quercetin supplementation or foods or drinks high in quercetin, such as apples and onions or black tea

- Rosemary

- Statin drugs that are used to lower cholesterol

- Thyroid medication if you are hypothyroid

Homocysteine

Homocysteine levels are commonly elevated in people with hypothyroidism. Homocysteine is an amino acid. High levels in the body induce endothelial dysfunction. This process is also one of the causes of oxidative stress which can lead to vascular disease and heart disease.

Oxidative stress is a term used to describe internal inflammation and the free radicals produced as a result of this inflammation. High homocysteine levels can damage the arterial lining of the heart, making it narrow and inelastic, a condition also known as "hardening" of the arteries (arteriosclerosis). When levels are elevated, homocysteine can also reduce nitric oxide production, which can lead to high blood pressure which is also a risk factor for heart disease. Furthermore, some researchers believe that high homocysteine levels also increase the risk of blood clotting which decreases blood flow through the arteries. One study showed that women with a history of high blood pressure and elevated homocysteine levels were twenty-five times more likely to have a heart attack or stroke than women whose blood pressure and homocysteine levels were closer to normal.

Lastly, if homocysteine levels are high this is usually reflective of decreased methylation in the body which increases your risk of not only heart disease but other diseases as well.

Causes of Elevated Levels

The following are causes of high homocysteine:

- Medications
- Hereditary predisposition
- Hypothyroidism
- Menopause
- Nutritional deficiencies of vitamins B6, B12, and folate
- Renal failure
- Smoking
- Toxins

In incidences where high homocysteine levels are hereditary, it is may be due to the fact that some people are lacking the enzyme methyltetrahydrofolate reductase, which breaks down homocysteine. A deficiency of this enzyme increases the need for a special type of folate (folic acid) in order to prevent high homocysteine levels. This occurs in at least 12 percent of the population of the United States. High homocysteine levels have been found to be associated with an increased risk in not just heart disease and stroke, but also osteoporosis, depression, memory loss, multiple sclerosis, type II diabetes, renal (kidney) failure, rheumatoid arthritis, and prostate and breast cancer.

Test Results

An optimal level of homocysteine is 6 to 8 micromoles/liter. Anything outside of this range should be addressed. Low levels can be just as dangerous as high levels.

Treatments

The following are ways to lower homocysteine levels:

- Exercise

- Increasing intake of broccoli, spinach, Brussels sprouts, cabbage, bok choy, or cauliflower (remember from Chapter 2 that too many of these vegetables can decrease the conversion of T4 to T3 and then negatively affect thyroid function, therefore use in moderation)

- Natural estrogen replacement therapy in patients that have low estrogen and are candidates for natural prescription estrogen replacement

- SAMe (s-adenosylmethionine), 200 to 400 mg a day

- Stress reduction

- Supplementation with vitamins B6, B12, folate or the activated form of folate, methyltetrahydrofolate, and the activated form of B6, which is pyridoxal-5-phosphate

- TMG (trimethylglycine) 400 to 500 mg twice a day

Researchers have suggested that folate supplementation could save 20,000 to 50,000 lives from heart disease every year.

Low TSH and High T4

Low TSH and higher T4 are associated with improved insulin sensitivity, higher HDL (good cholesterol), and better endothelial function. One study found that alterations in gene expression are reversible after restoring normal T3 plasma levels by giving T3. Since the heart is very vulnerable to a reduction in free T3, thyroid hormone replacement therapy with a combination of T3 and T4 has been found to be helpful to prevent and treat heart disease.

HYPERTHYROIDISM AND YOUR HEART

Hyperthyroidism can also lead to a number of complications in the body. It can directly alter the normal workings of the heart and vascular system causing serious complications. For patients with an overactive thyroid as seen in hyperthyroidism, existing cardiac symptoms can worsen or it can cause new ones in healthy hearts. It is essential that this thyroid condition be identified and treated correctly in order to prevent heart disease or to decrease cardiovascular symptoms. See Chapter 3 for more details on hyperthyroidism, on page 43.

SIGNS AND SYMPTOMS

There are many cardiovascular symptoms of hyperthyroidism that you should be aware of, such as the following:

❏ Chest pain related to the heart (angina)

❏ Exercise intolerance

❏ High blood pressure (systolic hypertension)

❏ Increased cardiac output

❏ Irregular heartbeat (atrial fibrillation)

❏ Palpitations, increased heart rate (tachycardia)

❏ Pulmonary hypertension

❏ Shortness of breath

❏ Swelling of the extremities (edema)

❏ Wide pulse pressure due to the increase in systolic and decease in diastolic pressure due to reduced resistance, lower resistance is due to an increase in nitric oxide production

HYPERTHYROIDISM AND CARDIOVASCULAR COMPLICATIONS

If hyperthyroidism is left untreated, it can lead to other health problems, such as cardiovascular or heart issues. The following are specific heart signs that your physician may find if you have hyperthyroidism.

Cardiac hypertrophy. When your heart has to pump harder in order to deliver blood to the rest of your body it may result in an enlarged heart. An enlarged heart may be associated with an overactive thyroid.

Congestive Heart Failure. When your heart is not able to pump blood to the organs of the body adequately and meet the demands placed on it, you may be suffering from congestive heart failure. In many cases alterations in thyroid hormone metabolism accompanies congestive heart failure. Congestive heart failure usually occurs in individuals that already have underlying heart disease and not as much in people that were young and healthy before they developed hyperthyroidism.

Inotropic effect. An inotropic effect can be applied to the conditions that alter the force of muscular contraction. Thyroid hormone production in excessive amounts has a direct inotropic effect on the heart muscle and cardiac contraction.

Irregular Heart Sounds. Irregular heart sounds may be enhanced and a scratchy systolic sound along the left sternal border may be present. When normal metabolic rate is restored, the symptoms and signs usually resolve.

Mitral Valve Prolapse. Mitral valve prolapse is a condition in which the two valve flaps of the mitral valve, during contraction, do not close evenly. This condition may result in a heart murmur. Mitral valve prolapse occurs more commonly in Grave's disease or Hashimoto's thyroiditis than in the general population.

Peripheral Resistance. Peripheral resistance is the exertion against the blood flow in the body. When the patient is at rest, the peripheral resistance is decreased and the cardiac output is increased. Hyperthyroidism results in a high output of the thyroid hormone and this hormone induced effect decreases the total peripheral resistance. The heart reacts to the low peripheral resistance by increasing in the heart rate. If left untreated an elevation in heart rate can increase the risk of developing a stroke.

Systolic and Diastolic Pressure. Your blood pressure readings are an indication of the amount of force or pressure that blood exerts on the blood vessels as it moves through. The systolic number (top) measures the amount of pressure the blood wields while the heart is beating. The diastolic number (bottom) measures the pressure in your vessels between heartbeats. These numbers can be affected by your hormone levels. An overactive thyroid can lead to high systolic blood pressure.

Heart (cardiac) output may be increased as much as 50 to 300 percent due to the combined effect of increased resting heart rate, increased con-

Hyperthyroidism in People Over 60

Irregular heart rhythm (atrial fibrillation) occurs in 10 to 15 percent of hyperthyroid patients of which most are 60 and older. Restoring normal heart rhythm is necessary since they are at an increased risk for blood clots (thromboembolic events), particularly if they already have a history of heart disease, high blood pressure, or previous blood clots or pulmonary embolism.

Likewise, subclinical hyperthyroidism often manifests itself differently in elderly patients. Older patients with subclinical hyperthyroidism are also at increased risk of developing atrial fibrillation. The following are potential heart problems associated with subclinical hyperthyroidism in the elderly.

- Decreased large and small artery elasticity
- Impaired left ventricular diastolic filling
- Impaired systolic function during exercise
- Increased cardiac contractility
- Increased intraventricular septal thickness
- Increased left ventricular mass index
- Increased left ventricular posterior wall thickness
- Prolonged QT interval

A medical study showed an increased incidence of Alzheimer's disease and other forms of dementia in patients that were over the age of 55 that had subclinical hyperthyroidism. This was even more common in patients with positive thyroid antibodies. Also, long-term studies of older people with untreated subclinical hyperthyroidism showed an increased risk of developing heart disease and death from all causes. Therefore, it is imperative that subclinical hyperthyroidism be treated. Treatment has been shown to improve the following cardiac functions:

- Decrease in atrial and ventricular premature beats
- Decrease in heart rate
- Decrease in left ventricular posterior wall thickness at diastole
- Reduction in interventricular septum thickness
- Reduction in left ventricular mass index

tractility, increased flow of blood, increased blood volume, and decreased resistance the blood experiences as it circulates throughout the body (systemic vascular resistance). It is interesting that the cardiovascular symptoms and signs are independent of the cause of the hyperthyroidism. In individuals that have pulmonary hypertension and hyperthyroidism, it may be associated with right-sided heart failure. The symptoms are due to increased circulatory demands from hyper-metabolism and the need for the body to decrease the excess heat produced. These complications are generally reversible with appropriate treatment.

TREATMENT

The treatment for hyperthyroidism depends on the cause and severity of the symptoms (see page 51). Treatment of the hyperthyroidism usually returns cardiac function to normal. In fact, 60 percent of people who have atrial fibrillation convert without cardioconversion (a medical procedure slowing down a fast heart rate to a normal heart rate) procedure to normal heart rhythm after they are treated for their hyperthyroidism within 4 months. Consequently, younger people are not usually given a blood thinner if they have no history of underlying heart disease or history of a prior problem with blood clots. If the person does not convert their heart rhythm to a normal one by taking medication to improve their heart rhythm, then cardioconversion is usually very successful up to one year after the diagnosis of thyrotoxicosis.

AMIODARONE-INDUCED THYROID DYSFUNCTION

Amiodarone is a regularly prescribed medication used for heart rhythm dysfunction. It is 37 percent iodine by weight and has a half-life of one hundred days. Due to its iodine content and chemical structure, which is similar to thyroid hormone, it may cause thyroid abnormalities. The risk is greater if you have positive thyroid antibodies. Amiodarone-induced hypothyroidism (AIT) is more common in iodine-sufficient areas of the world. At first, TSH levels may be normal then the individual may become hypothyroid.

Amiodarone may also cause hyperthyroidism. Amiodarone-induced hyperthyroidism is more frequently found in iodine-deficient areas of the world. First symptoms of amiodarone-induced thyrotoxicosis may be a new onset or recurrence of ventricular irritability (irritability of the heart), return or worsening heart failure symptoms and/or changes in Coumadin (a blood thinner) dose requirements. Thyrotoxicosis induced by amiodarone has two forms:

- Type I AIT, which is more common in iodine-deficient areas and is associated with preexisting thyroid abnormalities.

- Type II AIT is destructive or subacute thyroiditis that occurs in people with no history of previous thyroid disease.

CONCLUSION

As you have seen in this chapter, there is an important relationship between a well-functioning thyroid gland and the state of your cardiovascular health—a relationship which gets more important as you grow older. Understanding what happens to your heart when your thyroid malfunctions can be a matter of life and death. By being aware of the signs, by having an annual check-up, and asking the right questions, you can add years to your life. Knowing what to do when your thyroid malfunctions is key. Additionally, optimal thyroid function requires adequate nutritional intake. Hopefully, the information in this chapter will provide you with the options you may be in search of.

9

Thyroid Hormones and Digestive Health

As you've already learned, every biological function relies on a healthy thyroid gland, and the digestive process is no exception. Although many factors, from overall health to day-to-day diet, can affect digestion, normal digestion cannot take place without a well-functioning thyroid that produces appropriate amounts of thyroid hormones. Moreover, the thyroid relies on digestive health to support its own functions.

This chapter first looks at the significant connection between the thyroid and the digestive tract and examines the common problems that can occur when either system is not functioning as it should. The chapter then explores several additional digestive problems that are related to the thyroid gland.

HOW THE THYROID AND THE DIGESTIVE TRACT INTERACT

If you've ever looked at a list of thyroid dysfunction symptoms (see Chapters 2 and 3), you've likely seen several digestive problems among them. This is because by affecting the rate of metabolism—the speed with which reactions occur within the body—the thyroid can have pronounced effects on the digestive process.

Hyperthyroidism

When the thyroid is overactive (hyperthyroidism), your entire body tends to run on "high." By speeding up the digestive process and peristalsis—the wave-like muscle contractions that move food through the digestive tract—hyperthyroidism tends to make the stools pass too quickly through the digestive tract. Normally, as the waste moves down the tract, a certain

Understanding the Gut

In recent years, it has become clear that a healthy digestive system is essential to overall well-being. Amazingly, the gut is home to up to 70 percent of your immune system. Although this system is complex and beyond the scope of this book. It is significantly influenced and assisted by the 100 trillion or so bacteria, also called flora, that inhabit the gut. Without the flora, your immune system would be compromised. Unfortunately, not all gut bacteria support a strong immune system and good health. Some of the bacteria are "good," and others are "bad." Good bacteria aid in the metabolism and absorption of nutrients and help them get into the bloodstream. Bad bacteria, on the other hand, can cause painful gas, bloating, and inflammation. Worse, studies show that these less-beneficial bacteria emit chemicals that can damage the intestinal lining, leading to leaky gut syndrome, a condition in which the lining of the small intestine becomes damaged and allows food particles, waste products, and toxins to "leak" into the bloodstream. As you'll learn on page 147, healthy gut bacteria is crucial to your well-being in another way. They assist the conversion of the thyroid hormone T4 to hormone T3. Since T3 has about five times the hormone "strength" of T4, this substance is vital for the regulation of all metabolic processes within the body.

The 4R Program

Since gastrointestinal health, a healthy gut, is crucial for your overall health, you may want to follow this 4R program which is sure to help you and your gut heal. In order to diagnose leaky gut syndrome, a Functional Medicine

amount of water is removed from the waste and absorbed into the large intestines, causing the stools to become firmer, but not so firm that they can't pass easily out of the body. But transit time affects the firmness of the stools. When the waste material moves more quickly than normal, very little water has a chance to be removed, causing the stools to remain loose. This condition is referred to as diarrhea.

Hypothyroidism

On the other hand, when the thyroid is underactive (hypothyroidism), all the processes in the body, including the digestive process, tend to slow physician can order the test to make the diagnosis and can also help with the treatment. The 4R program is usually: remove, replace, repopulate, and repair.

Remove: Removing the source of the imbalance is the critical first step, be it pathogenic organisms or foods you are allergic to.

Replace: Replacing with hydrochloric acid, digestive enzymes, and herbal therapies is also very important. Acid is very important in the body. It has many functions including sterilizing the food you eat, and increasing the denaturing of proteins which prepares the protein for breakdown by gastric and pancreatic enzymes.

Repopulate: It is important that your GI tract be repopulated with healthy bacteria. Probiotics are microbial food supplements that beneficially affect your body by improving the intestinal microbal balance. Common probiotics are lactobacilli, bifidobactria, and saccharomyces.

Repair: There are nutrients that help the GI tract repair itself. Glutamine is an excellent nutrient that works on the small intestine. Glutamine stimulates the intestinal mucosal growth and protects against mucosal atrophy and plays an important role in acid-base balance in the body. Fasting has also been shown to be helpful in treating leaky gut syndrome. During fasting the white blood cell activity in the body increases which more effectively removes circulating immune complexes from the body and decreases inflammation and leaky gut syndrome. Herbal therapies such as Quercetin which is found in onions and blue-green algae has also been shown clinically to treat leaky gut syndrome.

down. When waste moves through the digestive tract too slowly, with the body absorbing more and more water along the way, the stools become hard and dry, and passing them becomes difficult and painful. This condition is referred to as constipation.

A Healthy Gut

You've now seen how an overactive or underactive thyroid can affect the bowel. But the bowel (or gut) can also have an effect on the function of the thyroid gland. You may remember from Chapter 1 that the thyroid produces more of the T4 hormone than the T3. It then relies on other organs and body systems to convert T4 into T3. About 20 percent of this conversion takes place in the gut. Scientists don't know the precise chain of events that allow this vital conversion to take place, but they have found that healthy gut flora ("good" bacteria) aid the conversions of T4 to T3. (To learn more about gut bacteria, see the inset on page 151.) Bad bacteria, however, may result in thyroid levels that are not as high as they should be. So the thyroid needs the gut just as the gut needs the thyroid.

The interaction between the gut and the thyroid is complex. For instance, the gut must be healthy enough to absorb the nutrients needed by the thyroid to do its job. If the digestive system is experiencing inflammation and can't absorb the nutrients iodine and selenium, both of which are crucial to thyroid function, the production of T3 and T4 will be reduced, and the metabolism—including digestive function—will slow.

If you are experiencing digestive problems that are not responding to treatment, it makes sense to get your thyroid function checked. Resolving any thyroid issues can be an essential part of restoring normal digestive function. Similarly, you'll want to make sure to safeguard your digestive health so that your thyroid is able to get the support its needs.

ACID REFLUX DISEASE

Patients with hypothyroidism (an insufficient production of thyroid hormones) often take antacids because they experience acid reflux, a condition in which the acidic gastric fluid flows up from the stomach into the esophagus, causing a burning chest pain called heartburn. If these symptoms occur more than twice a week, the disorder is called acid reflux disease or gastroesophageal reflex disease (GERD).

How Hypothyroidism Affects the Esophagus

To understand what is happening, you have to know a little about digestive physiology. A long muscular tube called the esophagus connects the stomach to the throat. Normally, a ring-shaped sphincter muscle called the lower esophageal sphincter (LES)—found at the lowest part of the esophagus, where the tube meets the stomach—prevents the acids in the stomach, as well as other stomach contents, from moving up the esophagus into the throat. (See Figure 8.1 on page 149.) But when someone is hypothyroid, both this sphincter and the one at the top of the esophagus (known as the upper esophageal sphincter, or UES) become lax and don't close properly. This enables the stomach contents—including stomach acids—to flow upwards into the esophagus. Because hypothyroidism slows the speed at which all activities in the body take place, it has been shown to delay gastric emptying which means that there is more acid present to flow into the esophagus. In addition to heartburn, symptoms of acid reflux can include chest pain, difficulty breathing, difficulty swallowing, hoarseness, sore throat, a dry cough, and the regurgitation of food or a sour liquid.

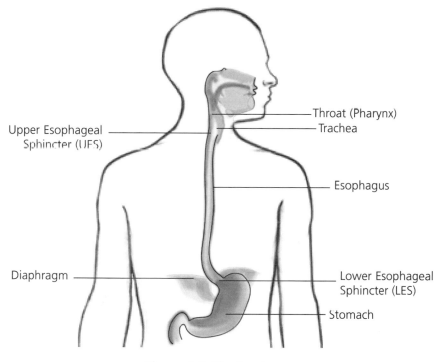

Figure 9.1. The Esophagus

Treatment

Believing that the stomach is producing too much stomach acid, hypothyroid patients often take antacids. Unfortunately, this approach does not always help, as the problem isn't always an overproduction of acid. In fact, hypothyroid patients are often found to be abnormally low in the hormone gastrin, which stimulates the secretion of gastric acid, and to also have lower levels of stomach acid than healthy people. By further lowering the acid in the stomach, antacids and other medications can create an environment in which food is not properly broken down and absorbed, and nutrient deficiencies—including deficiencies of the nutrients needed for the production of thyroid hormones—result. Moreover, levothyroxine, a medication used to treat hypothyroidism, requires stomach acid to become a bioidentical form of the thyroid hormone T4. If you have low stomach acid, either because of hypothyroidism or because of antacids, may find that this medication may not be as beneficial as it could be.

HELICOBACTER PYLORI (H. PYLORI)

For some people with hypothyroidism, heartburn may be caused or exacerbated by an infection of *Helicobacter pylori*, or *H. pylori*, the most common chronic bacterial pathogen found in human beings. Researchers are not sure of the mechanism that causes so many people with hypothyroidism to have *H. pylori* infections.

Helicobacter pylori and Hypothyroidism

Some studies have indicated that this bacteria may trigger autoimmune disorders such as Hashimoto's disease, the most common cause of hypothyroidism in the United States. Certainly, more people with Hashimoto's disease are affected by *H. pylori* than people in the general population. It is also known that acid-reducing medications, which are often taken by people with hypothyroidism, create an ideal condition for *H. pylori* to thrive. One five-year study published in *The New England Journal of Medicine* found that rates of *H. pylori* increased from 59 percent to 81 percent in patients taking one over-the-counter acid-reducing medication. Heartburn is just one possible symptom associated with these bacteria. Other symptoms, ranging from bloating to burning abdominal pain, may also be present. (See the inset on page 151 to learn more about *Helicobacter pylori* bacteria.)

Treatment

The good news is that the acid reflux associated with hypothyroidism can often be relieved. When thyroid hormone is used to treat hypothyroidism and levels of T3 and T4 are returned to normal, appropriate tension of the lower esophageal sphincter is usually restored. This prevents stomach

Helicobacter Pylori—
An Underdiagnosed Digestive Villain

On page 150, you learned that *Helicobacter pylori*—a bacteria that can cause infection of the stomach—can result in heartburn and other digestive problems. You also learned that this is one of the most common infections worldwide, and that it is more common in people with thyroid dysfunction than it is in the general population. But despite its prevalence, it too often goes undiagnosed.

Part of the explanation for the under-recognition of *H. pylori* is the fact that in some people, it causes no symptoms. In these cases, the infection, which usually occurs because of food-borne bacteria or contaminated utensils, remains localized in the gastric area at so low a level that no one is aware of its presence. In other people, though, the bacteria can lead to a number of distressing problems, including abdominal pain, acid reflux, bloating, nausea, vomiting, loss of appetite, and loss of weight. Sometimes, these symptoms indicate serious disorders. *H. pylori* is, in fact, present in 60 to 100 percent of patients with gastric ulcers, and 90 to 100 percent of patients with duodenal ulcers. Moreover, it is associated with stomach cancer and lymphoma.

Because infection with *H. pylori* is so common, in the absence of symptoms, doctors often recommend no treatment whatsoever. But since this organism sometimes results in serious conditions, physicians are becoming increasingly interested in diagnosing and treating it. Several diagnostic tests are now available—endoscopy, a breath test, a blood test, and a very accurate fecal antigen test. Once diagnosed, an *H. pylori* infection is generally treated with a combination of antibiotics. In some cases the combination of zinc and the amino acid carnosine are also used to treat *H. pylori*.

If you are experiencing any of the symptoms of *H. pylori,* be sure to get tested for this common bacteria. If the test is positive, remember that this bacteria can have nasty consequences, so it pays to get prompt treatment.

acid from escaping into the esophagus. Treatment with thyroid hormone also causes the levels of gastrin and stomach acid to normalize. When *H. pylori* is the problem, antibiotics usually offer a solution, and heartburn disappears along with the infection.

If you are suffering from chronic acid reflux, keep in mind that this disorder is not always caused by the overproduction of stomach acids, and that antacids and similar medications may not be the answer. If you have been diagnosed with thyroid disease, you may find that correcting your thyroid dysfunction also soothes your digestive tract. People with thyroid disorders are seldom tested for *H. pylori* even when symptoms are present, so be sure that your physician considers all possible causes and their treatments.

CELIAC DISEASE

Another way in which thyroid disease is connected to digestive health is through the incidence of celiac disease. Celiac disease is an autoimmune disorder that manifests itself when people eat gluten, a protein found in wheat, barley, rye, and products made from these ingredients. When the gluten reaches the digestive tract, an immune response is triggered in the small intestine, causing symptoms that can include diarrhea, bloating, abdominal pain, and weight loss. Over time, this causes inflammation of the lining of the small intestine and prevents nutrients from being adequately absorbed, a condition known as malabsorption.

Celiac Disease and Thyroid Disease

A significant number of patients with celiac disease have autoimmune thyroid disease (ATD)—either Hashimoto's disease (a type of hypothyroidism) or Graves' disease (the most common form of hyperthyroidism). In fact, people with celiac disease are nearly 4 times more likely to develop an autoimmune thyroid condition than people who do not have celiac disease. The reverse also holds true: People with autoimmune thyroid disease are far more likely to develop celiac disease than the general public. In one study conducted by Dr. Alessio Fasano, a celiac disease researcher, half of the people newly diagnosed with celiac disease also had a dysfunctional thyroid.

So far, scientists aren't sure why the connection exists between autoimmune thyroid disease and celiac. Some have hypothesized that people with celiac disease and autoimmune thyroid disorders share a genetic predisposition. Some have observed that the anti-tTG antibodies which are present in people with active celiac disease also bind and react to thyroid tissue and may stimulate the development of ATD. Some health

Following a Gluten-Free Diet

As you learned on page 154, people who have an autoimmune thyroid disorder can often benefit from following a gluten-free diet. And, of course, anyone with celiac disease or gluten sensitivity *must* stick to gluten-free foods. The following gluten-containing grains and grain-based products need to be avoided on a gluten-free diet:

- Barley
- Bulgur wheat
- Couscous (usually made from wheat)
- Einkorn (a type of wheat)

- Kamut (a type of wheat)
- Pasta made from wheat, rye, or barley.
- Rye

- Semolina (the hard part of wheat)
- Spelt (a type of wheat)
- Triticale (a wheat hybrid)
- Wheat

The following grains and grain substitutes may be consumed on a gluten-free diet:

- Almond flour
- Amaranth
- Buckwheat
- Coconut flour

- Corn
- Cornstarch
- Millet
- Potato flour

- Quinoa
- Rice (white, brown, and wild)
- Sorghum
- Teff

In addition to avoiding gluten-containing grains and flours, it is essential to become aware of processed products that contain ingredients made from these grains. Most soy sauce, for instance, is made with fermented wheat, so you'll need to look for a gluten-free brand. Many sauces and soups and some condiments—even some types of ketchup and mustard—use gluten-based thickeners. Since naturally gluten-free, oats often become cross-contaminated during processing, you'll need to search out brands that are made for people who can't have gluten. Read food package labels carefully for statements about gluten, and if in doubt, contact the manufacturer for more information.

care providers believe that in a number of people who develop Hashimoto's, the thyroid disease is triggered by underlying celiac disease or gluten sensitivity. Whatever the mechanism involved— the connection between autoimmune thyroid disease and celiac disease has been well established by study after study.

Treatment

Fortunately, just as thyroid autoimmune disease and celiac disease are interrelated, a similar method of management appears to offer relief to people with both disorders. A gluten-free diet is essential to people with celiac disease and gluten sensitivity. When people with celiac follow this diet, their anti-tTG antibodies—which indicate that the disease is present and active—decrease and may eventually disappear. When people with ATD follow a gluten-free diet, their thyroid antibody levels have also been found to decrease. In some cases, when people with both celiac and Hashimoto's have followed a gluten-free diet, thyroid function has returned to normal and the individuals have no longer needed thyroid medication. Although this type of complete recovery is rare— usually, autoimmune diseases require lifelong treatment—many clinicians have stated that a gluten-free diet is essential for those with this form of ATD.

If you have an autoimmune thyroid disease—Hashimoto's or Graves'—it is important to be tested for celiac disease. People with celiac do not always experience digestive upset, especially at the onset on the disease, so even if you feel that your digestion is working well, a test for celiac may be able to provide more information about your condition. Considering the evidence, it also makes sense to try a gluten-free diet. (See the inset on page 153.) For most people with ATD, excluding gluten has proven essential to help optimize their thyroid function.

CONCLUSION

If you have been diagnosed with hypothyroidism or hyperthyroidism, it is paramount that you get the treatment you need. This alone may relieve your digestive problems. If you have not been diagnosed with thyroid dysfunction but are experiencing one or more digestive issues, be aware that thyroid disorders are a common cause and should be considered. Also recognize that a range of other issues, such as infection by *H. pylori* bacteria, can cause GI problems. By understanding the potential culprits, you'll be better prepared to search for the cause of your digestive disorder.

Sometimes, it is necessary to use a combination of treatments to experience optimal digestive health. For instance, to resolve issues such as diarrhea or constipation, you may need to pair treatment for thyroid dysfunction with a healthier diet and/or probiotics. By using a treatment program developed by a qualified physician who is aware of all your medical issues, you can enhance thyroid function, improve your digestion, and safeguard your overall health.

10

Thyroid Cancer

The number of thyroid cancer cases have more than doubled since the early 1970s, and for women, it is the cancer with the fastest-growing number of new cases. As of 2015, the incidence of thyroid cancer is estimated to be 62,450 cases in the US. It currently stands as the fifth most common cancer in women. And like most other thyroid diseases, it occurs approximately 3 times more often in women than in men. While that may sound frightening, the overall odds of beating the majority of thyroid cancers are in your favor. So the more you know, the better prepared you will be to understand what it is, and how, in most cases, it can be successfully treated.

It is, however, important to also point out that just finding a nodule on the thyroid gland does not mean the growth is malignant. Each year there are over 1.2 million patients who are diagnosed with thyroid nodules. Many of these nodules are ruled out as benign using an ultrasound scan. Of the 525,000 to 600,000 nodules that are biopsied every year, only 10 percent are found to be malignant.

Still, knowledge is power, so this chapter has been designed to provide you with not only an understanding of the most common terms related to thyroid cancer, but also an overview of the entire process. It begins by looking at what thyroid cancer is then examines the risk factors involved, its many signs and symptoms, and the tests used to determine if it is thyroid cancer. Once test results come back, there will be descriptive terms used that patients need to understand. Explained are the most common terms under the sections on visual characteristics of thyroid cancer cells, its stages, and the standard treatments available. This is followed by a discussion concerning each type of thyroid cancer. The chapter concludes with practical suggestions patients should consider when preparing for what's ahead of them.

WHAT IS THYROID CANCER?

As discussed in Chapter 1, the thyroid gland is composed of several types of cells. This includes the follicular cells, the parafollicular cells (C cells), and the endothelial cells. When a clump of cells unexpectedly begins to grow in the thyroid, they may be either benign (non-cancerous) or malignant (cancerous). Benign growths tend to grow slowly and stop at a certain point; malignant growths, on the other hand, contain cells that begin to multiply uncontrollably and can spread to nearby tissues as well as other parts of the body. Tumors that have spread to other parts of the body are called metastasis. It is important to know that some thyroid cancers may grow very slowly and go undetected for years.

The type of thyroid cancer that may occur is based on the specific thyroid cell that has become malignant. Therefore, quickly learning what type of thyroid cancer the tumor is composed of is very important since the odds of success are based on the make-up of the thyroid cancer. It is also important to know that some thyroid tumors can be composed of more than one type of malignant thyroid cell as well as benign cells. The good news is that the overall 5-year survival rate of patients with the most common thyroid cancer is 98 percent. We will learn more about the survival rates as we discuss the various types of thyroid cancers.

RISK FACTORS

While anyone may be susceptible to developing thyroid cancer, there are those who may be at a higher risk based upon the following risk factors:

Family History

Certain genes can be passed on from one generation to the next which can greatly increase the odds of developing the thyroid cancer. It has been found that where there is a family history of precancerous polyps in the colon or goiters, the risk of papillary thyroid cancer increases. In addition, specific medullary thyroid cancer-prone genes can be passed on as well.

Radiation Exposure

During the 1950s, children were treated using radiation therapy for non-cancerous conditions, such as enlarged thymus, acne, ringworm, or enlargement of the tonsils or adenoids, and currently children who have had imaging tests such as x-rays and CT scans or have undergone certain radiation treatments may have a higher risk of developing thyroid cancer. Similar exposure by adults may also increase the odds of their having this disease. In addition, anyone who has been exposed to radiation from power plant accidents or nuclear fallout may also be at greater risk of developing thyroid cancer.

Age and Gender

While thyroid cancer can develop in people who are in their 20s and up, statistics indicate that women in their 40s and 50s are 3 times more likely to develop thyroid cancer than men. For men, they are at greater risk in their 60s and 70s.

Iodine Intake

A lack of iodine in one's diet can lead to enlargement of the thyroid and mental retardation in infants and children. In addition, low iodine intake can increase the odds of developing follicular cancer and papillary cancer (with radiation exposure). Usually, the standard western diet provides a sufficient level of iodine through intake of iodized salt and other foods. Studies have also shown that excessive iodine supplementation may be linked to an increase in developing thyroid cancer.

Race

Statistics indicated that Caucasian and Asian people are more likely to develop thyroid cancer, however it is important to point out that no one group is exempt. For example, while the black population shows the lowest rates of thyroid cancer among any groups, the greatest rate of papillary thyroid cancer acceleration has been recorded in black females.

Still, while statistics may show a person's level of risk may be on the high side, any adult can be at risk; it is important for all of us to become aware of the signs and symptoms of thyroid cancer.

SIGN AND SYMPTOMS

A number of the physical warning signs of thyroid cancer can provide us with an opportunity to catch it in an early stage. The following are the most common symptoms:

❑ **Swollen lymph nodes.** Normally, a swollen lymph gland is a sign of infection; however, it may also be the site of a thyroid cancer tumor.

❑ **Lump in the neck.** A new lump appearing in front of the Adam's apple or to either side may be an indication.

❑ **Pain in the throat or neck.** Unexplained pain in the throat or neck may be due to an enlargement of the neck caused by swollen lymph nodes or a tumor pressing against the trachea (windpipe) or esophagus.

❑ **Hoarseness.** Changes in your voice or a persistent hoarseness may be due to pressure from an enlarged thyroid gland or a growth which sits just beneath the larynx (voice box).

❑ **Difficulty swallowing.** Unexplained pain when swallowing food may be caused by an enlargement of the neck or a tumor pressing against the trachea which sits above the esophagus.

❑ **Trouble breathing.** Breathing difficulty may be caused by an enlargement of the neck or a tumor pressing against the trachea which sits above the esophagus.

❑ **Wheezing.** Unexplained wheezing may be caused by an enlargement of the neck or a tumor pressing against the trachea.

❑ **Persistent cough.** A cough that is not due to a cold may be caused by an enlargement of the neck or a tumor pushing against the larynx or trachea.

If any of these warning signs appear, without any recent history of infections, it would be wise to see a physician immediately to determine the cause of the problem. A toothache, a sinus infection, or a benign growth can mimic the signs of a cancerous nodule. However, the quicker the cause is found, the quicker the right treatment can be applied.

Unfortunately, there are times thyroid cancer progresses without any early symptoms. Instead, the only signs and symptoms to appear occur when the thyroid cancer tumors interfere with the thyroid's normal regulation of life functions—from problems with weight to blood pressure to heart rate. The underlying problem can only be discovered through a thorough physical examination by a doctor who can perform or recommend several possible tests.

TESTING FOR THYROID CANCER

If the initial signs indicate a possible thyroid problem, there are a number of tests health care providers may offer patients to determine if they have thyroid cancer, and if they do, what type of thyroid cancer it is. The most common are:

Thyroid Ultrasound

Sound waves are used to create a visual image of the thyroid. This is done when a small wand-like instrument is moved along the skin in front of the thyroid gland. The black and white image seen on a computer screen will show whether the node is composed of a solid mass of cells or a cyst containing blood or pus. If it is a solid node, further testing needs to be done to determine if the mass is benign or cancerous.

Fine Needle Aspiration (FNA)

If the node is found to be solid, a fine-needle aspiration is taken. The skin above the node is numbed, and a thin needle is inserted into the node to remove cells and fluid for review. These samples are then sent to a laboratory where a pathologist examines them under a microscope to determine the exact nature of the cells. The pathologist writes up a report on his/her findings and sends back the report to the ordering doctor.

While the FNA is designed to determine if the cells are benign or cancerous, up to 30 percent of the FNA biopsy may be inconclusive. In many cases another FNA is taken, however due to the type of thyroid cancer it may be, the results may still be inconclusive. When this happens a blood test may be able to provide an answer. However, should it not, traditionally, surgery is the next step to determine if the node is benign or cancerous. Recently, however, a new personalized genetic test has been developed to provide an answer based on the initial FNA biopsy, which can prevent unnecessary surgeries. (See Personalized Genetic Test below.)

Personalized Genetic Test

Beyond just testing for inherited thyroid cancer-prone genes, there are new personalized genetic tests available which may be able to rule out whether the cells taken from a FNA procedure are benign or malignant. Additionally, the test may determine how aggressive a BRAF (a genetic alteration) gene-based thyroid cancer cell may be. These tests are based upon molecular identification. The results of such tests can enable a surgeon to determine how extensive a surgery is needed or if one is required at all.

Blood Calcitonin Test

Calcitonin is a hormone produced by the parafollicular cells, also known as C-cell, found in the thyroid. It acts to reduce calcium found in the blood. When the amount of calcitonin in the blood is found to be high, it can indicate the presence of C-cell hyperplasia, a pre-cancerous stage which may lead to medullary thyroid cancer. However, C-cell hyperplasia, in and of itself, is a benign condition. This blood test may be ordered when any of the risk factors described above are present.

Radioiodine Thyroid Scan

Unlike the thyroid ultrasound, the thyroid scan requires a radioactive iodine tracer be swallowed or injected into the blood stream. The signals given off by the radiation can measure how much tracer is absorbed from the blood and the scan itself can show the location, shape, and size of the gland as well as nodules that may be located within the gland.

Computed Tomography (CT)

A CT scan is a computerized x-ray that shows a detailed cross-sectional image of the thyroid and its surrounding area. It requires that a contrast solution be swallowed or given through an IV line. The solution contains a dye which outlines the thyroid gland along with any mass and structure within the neck area.

Magnetic Resonance Imaging (MRI)

Just like the CT scan, the MRI scan shows a more detailed cross-section of the thyroid and its surrounding area. Instead of x-rays, it uses radio waves and magnets to create its images. A contrasting solution is injected in the blood stream and the dye outlines the thyroid gland along with any mass and structure within the neck area.

Positron Emission Tomography (PET) Scan

A PET scan can produce a three-dimensional image using gamma rays. A substance containing a radioactive form of sugar is injected into the blood stream. The radioactive sugar is quickly absorbed by tumors which will show up in its images. While not as finely detailed as CT or MRI scans, PET scans can provide a full body image of possible cancer sites.

VISUAL CHARACTERISTICS OF THYROID CANCERS CELLS

As we will see, the different kinds of thyroid cancers stem from specific types of thyroid cells. There are a number of important terms that are associated with the way these cancer cells appear. These terms are commonly used in pathology reports to provide a physician with a detailed picture of the type of cells contained in a tumor.

Differentiated cancer cells. While some cancer cells may look and behave like normal cells, others may change their appearance. Under a microscope, all their internal structures are clearly identifiable. Like normal thyroid cells, they absorb iodine; however, unlike normal cells these cancer cells will grow unregulated and may spread.

Poorly differentiated cancer cells. Under a microscope, these cells may be missing certain internal structures or their internal structures are malformed. In some cases, there are enough functioning structures within the cell to identify the type of thyroid cell it originates from. However, sometimes identifying the origin of these cells is difficult. In some cases, they may also lack the ability to absorb iodine.

Undifferentiated cancer cells. Although these cells may originate from a specific thyroid cell, they do not contain enough internal structures to be linked to a specific type of thyroid cell. And unlike other thyroid cancer cells, they lack the ability to absorb iodine.

Encapsulated tumor. This refers to a cancerous growth that is completely surrounded by benign cells. Once the tumor has been removed, the pathologist will determine whether it is encapsulated. This type of tumor will influence the follow-up treatments.

Margins. Margins refer to the outer edges of a tumor. When hair-like structures extend outward from the surface, this is called positive margins. When there are no hair-like structures, this is called negative margins. When there is limited growth of these extensions, it is called close margins. During the surgical removal of a tumor, it is difficult for the surgeon to determine the type of margins present since some of these growths may be microscopic in size. Once the tumor has been removed, the pathologist will determine whether it is positive, negative, or close. The type of margin found will influence the follow-up treatments.

Mixture of thyroid cancer cells. A number of times pathology reports find different types of cells within a single tumor. The findings may show benign cells with a mix of one or two cancerous types. Treatments for these types of tumors may range widely: from treatments designed to combat the most aggressive thyroid cancer first to prescribing several treatments at once to fight all the cancers.

Tumor size. Tumors are measures in centimeters (cm). A 1cm is a little smaller than a $1/2$-inch; 3cm is a little bigger than an 1-inch; and 5cm is a little smaller than 2-inches. The size of a tumor may determine the treatment given.

STAGES OF THYROID CANCER

In general, all cancers are classified in terms of how far the cancer has spread. Normally, the location(s), the size of tumors, and the patient's age may determine the stage at which a cancer has progressed. In some cases, however, the speed at which a cancer may progress determines its stage. All thyroid cancers have their own specific stages; however, as a general rule of thumb the following factors determine a thyroid cancer's stage.

Stage 0. This refers to an early stage of medullary thyroid cancer in which a specialized screening test indicates the presents of medullary cells with no physical thyroid tumor being detected.

Stage I. The tumor is found inside of the thyroid with or without limited spread to nearby tissues and lymph nodes.

Stage II. The tumor is found inside the thyroid and has metastasized to other parts of the body. The tumor itself is small, 2cm in size or smaller.

Stage III. The tumor is found inside the thyroid and has metastasized to other parts of the body. The tumor may be 2cm to 4cm in size or greater.

Stage IV. The tumor is found inside the thyroid and is now wide-spread throughout the body. However, in the case of anaplastic and undifferentiated thyroid cancer, any finding of this type of cancer is immediately classified as stage IV whether or not it has spread.

STANDARD TREATMENTS

Each type of thyroid cancer has its own treatment steps called protocols. While these protocols may differ in duration, sequence, and/or dosage based upon the individual patients, the following treatments are most common.

Surgery

In a *lobectomy,* only the side containing the tumor is removed. In a *partial thyroidectomy,* the majority of the thyroid is removed leaving only a small section in place. In a *total thyroidectomy* the entire thyroid is taken out. If there is evidence that any of the nearby lymph nodes contain cancer cells, a *lymph node dissection* is performed.

Radioactive Iodine (RAI)

For those cancer thyroid cells that continue to absorb iodine, this treatment can be highly effective. Radioactive iodine is swallowed in a liquid form or capsule. The RAI is then absorbed into all the functioning thyroid cells. As the RAI is collected within the cells, the concentration of radiation destroys the thyroid gland along with the cancerous cell.

Radiation Therapy

High energy x-rays are focused on a general area of the neck using any number of external radiation machines. In some cases, a small dosage of chemotherapy is given to the patient to enhance the effect of the radiation. This treatment is designed to kill cancer cells and shrink tumors.

Chemotherapy

Chemotherapeutic agents are anti-cancer drugs that may be taken by mouth or injection. These medications are given to kill or shrink tumors. Based on the specific chemo, there may be a number of side effects with some becoming so intense that the chemotherapy must be stopped. Some of the side effects may be short-lived while others may be permanent.

Radiation and Chemotherapy

In some case, before the radiation session begins, a low dosage of chemo is given to the patient to enhance the effect of the radiation. In other cases, a full dosage of chemo is given along with the radiation treatments. This type of combination is considered aggressive.

Targeted Drugs

The FDA has approved a number of drugs specifically designed to combat various thyroid cancers. They work on the basis of disrupting the cancer cells' ability to function. Some do this by cutting off the tumor's blood supply, by interfering with its internal pathways, or by attaching chemicals to its receptors. Some of these drugs are used in conjunction with certain chemotherapies. While still in the early stages, these drugs provide a new weapon against these malignancies.

Clinical Trials

In many medical centers, clinical trials of new and unproven treatments are offered for free to patients who have met certain criteria—perhaps having exhausted all other standard treatments. These clinical trials may include new drugs, new chemotherapies, or a combination of drugs and/or chemotherapeutic agents.

There are four phases of a clinical trial:

- **Phase I** evaluates a treatment for its safety and the best way it can be administered

- **Phase II** determines which cancer it works best against

- **Phase III** measures its effectiveness compared to similar FDA approved treatments

- **Phase IV** studies the effect of its long–term use as well as its side effects

Before entering any clinical trial, it is wise to ask what phase the trial is in, and what the preliminary results of the trials have shown.

Hormone Therapy

Once the thyroid gland has been fully or partially removed, the drug levothyroxine sodium will be prescribed. This is a synthetic compound identical to the thyroid hormone T4 (levothyroxine). In addition to replacing the hormones normally made by the thyroid gland, it acts to suppress the TSH levels to reduce the chance of the cancer from recurring.

TYPES OF THYROID CANCERS

Once the type of thyroid cancer has been determined, you may see either an endocrinologist, a doctor specializing in thyroid disorders, and/or an oncologist, a doctor specializing in cancer. With rare and/or aggressive cancers, you would most likely be treated by an oncologist; otherwise the cancer is usually treated by an endocrinologist. Normally, cancers of the thyroid that are differentiated are very treatable and commonly curable. Tumors that are poorly differentiated are more aggressive and normally require more intensive treatments. The following information will provide a description of the individual types of thyroid cancers as well as their treatments. Some treatments for the same cancers differ based on a patient's age.

PAPILLARY THYROID CANCER
(PAPILLARY THYROID CARCINOMA)

Papillary thyroid cancer cells originate from the uncontrolled growth of follicular cells. It is referred to as a carcinoma since it begins in the tissue lining the inner or outer surface of the thyroid. This represents approximately 70 to 80 percent of all thyroid cancers, making it the most common form. The vast majority of papillary cancer cells are differentiated.

There are, however, some rare but aggressive variant forms of papillary cancer cells. These include tall cell, columnar cell, diffuse sclerosing variant (DSV), and hobnail variant. They are poorly differentiated. These cells may be mixed in with the differentiated papillary thyroid cancer cells.

Potential Spread

It can spread to the surrounding tissues and lymph nodes. These additional growths in the neck area are called cervical metastasis. Although uncommon, it can spread to the lungs and bones.

Tests

Blood tests, ultrasound, scans, a fine needle aspiration (FNA), and/or a personalized genetic test may be performed.

Treatments

Surgery. Surgery is normally first done to remove the tumor(s). This may require removal of one side of the thyroid gland or the complete thyroid. When surgery cannot be done, the patient may receive radiation therapy.

Radioactive iodine. After surgery, radioactive iodine (RAI) is given.

External beam radiation therapy. This therapy may be offered to kill those papillary cancer cells that were not eradicated by the RAI treatment.

Levothyroxine sodium. Once the treatments have been completed, patients will normally be required to take the drug levothyroxine sodium, a synthetic thyroid hormone, for the rest of their lives.

Blood tests. Follow-up blood tests are normally given every 6 to 12 months to check on thyroid hormone levels.

OUTCOMES (PROGNOSIS)

The survival rate for this type of cancer is good with more than 95 percent of adults having a survival rate of at least 10 years. Having check-ups regularly to catch potential reoccurrence is very important since early detection greatly increases survival rates.

FOLLICULAR THYROID CANCER
(FOLLICULAR CARCINOMA)

Follicular thyroid cancer represents 10 to 15 percent of all cases of thyroid cancer. A follicular carcinoma develops from the uncontrolled growth of the follicular cell. As with papillary, it is well differentiated. There is also a benign form of this cell called a follicular adenoma which, in the past, could not be identified when compared to the follicular carcinoma in early tests. The new personalized genetic test may help determine if the follicular cell is malignant.

As with papillary cancer, the follicular cancer cell has its own form of variant cells. That variant form is Hurthle cell thyroid cancer. (See Hurthle Cell Cancer, page 170.)

Potential Spread

Usually follicular cancer does not spread to the surrounding tissue and lymph nodes. However, while some forms of follicular cancer are minimally invasive, others can be highly aggressive. When aggressive, these cells can spread to any and all organs throughout the body.

Tests

Early testing using blood tests, ultrasound, scans, and/or a fine needle aspiration (FNA) can identify the growth as coming from the follicular cell. A personalized genetic test may identify the cells as cancerous at an earlier stage; however, standard practice is to remove the tumor through surgery, and have it evaluated by a pathologist, so that the tumor can be accurately identified as follicular thyroid cancer.

Treatments

Surgery. Surgery is normally first done to remove the tumor(s). This may require removal of one side of the thyroid gland or the complete thyroid. Normally, the size of the growth and the patient's age may determine how much of the thyroid gland is removed. When surgery cannot be done, the patient may receive radiation therapy.

Radioactive iodine. After surgery, radioactive iodine (RAI) is given. Absorption of the RAI is enhanced by giving the patient high levels of thyroid-stimulating hormones (TSH).

External beam radiation therapy. Based on the extent of the tumor and the effect of RAI treatment on the follicular cancer cells, external beam radiation therapy may be offered to kill the remaining cancer cells.

Levothyroxine sodium. Once the treatment has been completed, patients will normally be required to take the drug levothyroxine sodium, a synthetic thyroid hormone, for the rest of their lives.

Blood tests. Follow-up blood tests are normally given every 6 to 12 months to check on thyroid hormone levels.

Outcomes (Prognosis)

The survival rate for this type of cancer is 90 percent when the follicular cells are differentiated, however, the recurrence rate can be as high as 30 percent. Having check-ups regularly to catch potential reoccurrence is very important since early detection greatly increases survival rates.

HURTHLE CELL THYROID CANCER
(HURTHLE CELL CARCINOMA)

Because Hurthle cell thyroid cancer is a variant form of follicular thyroid cell, it is classified under follicular thyroid cancer. Hurthle cell is considered a rare cancer, accounting for 5 to 10 percent of differentiated thyroid cancers. When a follicular cell turns into a Hurthle cell, it takes on a vastly different appearance. Unlike normal follicular cells, however, they do not provide a useful service to the body. Hurthle cells may be benign or malignant. Like the follicular growths, the benign form of this cell, called a Hurthle cell adenoma, has been hard to identify when compared to the Hurthle cell carcinoma in early tests. The new personalized genetic test may help determine if the follicular cell is malignant.

Hashimoto's thyroiditis or Hashimoto's disease, an inherited disorder, may increase the odds of developing Hurthle cells in the thyroid.

Potential Spread

Like follicular cancer, Hurthle cells do not usually spread to the surrounding tissue and lymph nodes. Some Hurthle cells can be minimally invasive, while others can be highly aggressive. When aggressive, these cells can spread to any and all organs throughout the body. While benign Hurthle cell tumors may not be dangerous, and do not usually grow back once removed, some of these benign cells may turn cancerous in rare instances.

Tests

Blood tests, ultrasound, scans, and/or a fine needle aspiration (FNA) can identify the growth as being Hurthle cell. A personalized genetic test may identify the cells as cancerous at an earlier stage; however, standard practice is to remove the tumor through surgery, have it evaluated by a pathologist, so that the tumor can be accurately identified as Hurthle cell.

Treatments

Surgery. Surgery is normally first done to remove the tumor(s). This may require removal of one side of the thyroid gland or the complete thyroid. Normally, the size of the growth and the patient's age may determine how much of the thyroid gland is removed. When surgery cannot be done, the patient may receive radiation therapy.

Radioactive iodine (RAI). After surgery, radioactive iodine (RAI) is given. Absorption of the RAI is enhanced by giving the patient high levels of thyroid-stimulating hormones (TSH).

External beam radiation therapy. Based on the extent of the tumor and the effect of RAI treatment on the Hurthle cells, external beam radiation therapy may be offered to kill the remaining cancer cells.

Levothyroxine sodium. Once the treatment has been completed, patients will normally be required to take the drug levothyroxine sodium, a synthetic thyroid hormone, for the rest of their lives.

Blood tests. Follow-up blood tests are normally given every 6 to 12 months to check on thyroid hormone levels.

Outcomes (Prognosis)

Statistics indicate that the survival rate for this type of cancer may be correlated to the age of the patient, the size of the tumor, how differentiated the cells are, and whether or not the tumor has metastasized. Usually, the younger the patient and smaller the tumor, the better the outcome. Older patients with metastasis may be at a disadvantage, however, in rare cancers such as this, survival rates are best evaluated on a case by case basis.

MEDULLARY THYROID CANCER
(MEDULLARY CARCINOMA)

Medullary thyroid cancer (MTC) originates from the parafollicular cells (also called C cells) of the thyroid. Though statistically low in numbers, they are the third most common thyroid cancer making up 3 to 10 percent percent of all thyroid cancers. This type of cancer cell is less differentiated than papillary and follicular.

Normal parafollicular cells secrete a number of hormones, including

calcitonin, ACTH, *serotonin, prostaglandins,* and vasoactive intestinal pep-
tide *(VIP).* When the parafollicular cells change into medullary cancer
cells, however, they produce larger and larger amounts of these hormones
as they increase in numbers. This may create several health issues, including high levels of calcitonin and diarrhea.

There are two types of medullary thyroid cancers: One is *sporadic MTC*
which does not run in families and the second is *inherited MTC.* Sporadic
MTC accounts for 75 to 80 percent of all medullary thyroid cancers. Inherited MTC, which accounts for the remaining 20 to 25 percent, may include
a group of other endocrine disorders. These disorders may become evident
in a variety of symptoms associated with each affected endocrine gland.

Potential Spread

Initially, medullary tumors tend to be located in the back of the thyroid
gland, closer to the larynx and trachea. Therefore as it grows it may commonly compress or invade the throat area resulting in hoarseness or respiratory difficulty. It may also spread to nearby lymph nodes. While there
may be a lower percentage of metastasis spreading to other parts of the
body, when it does occur, the common areas include the chest cavity, liver,
lungs, and bones.

Tests

Blood tests, ultrasound, scans, a fine needle aspiration (FNA), and/or personalized genetic test may be performed.

Treatments

Surgery. Surgery is normally first done to remove the tumor(s). This may
require removal of one side of the thyroid gland or the complete thyroid
based upon the tumor's involvement with the structures around it.

Radioactive iodine (RAI). After surgery, radioactive iodine (RAI) is usually not given. Because the medullary cell does not readily absorb iodine,
RAI has little effect on this type of thyroid cancer.

External beam radiation therapy. External beam radiation may be uti-
lized, however the use of it must be based on the individual case.

Chemotherapy. Standard chemotherapy may be an option, however such
treatments have shown limited effectiveness.

Drugs. There are a number of new targeted drugs available that are aimed at blocking the pathways necessary to the development and progression of medullary cancer cells. You can learn more about these drugs from your oncologist.

Levothyroxine sodium. Once the treatment has been completed, patients will normally be required to take the drug levothyroxine sodium, a synthetic thyroid hormone, for the rest of their lives.

Blood tests. Follow-up blood tests are normally given every 6 to 12 months to check on thyroid hormone levels.

Outcomes (Prognosis)

Patients with disease limited to only the thyroid gland, without nodal involvement, have a very low risk for recurrence and rarely die from their disease. However, patents with nodal involvement are at a higher risk for recurrence or persistent disease. Overall, however, the outcome for patients with MTC is good. The 10-year survival rate for MTC patients is 75 to 85 percent.

ANAPLASTIC THYROID CANCER AND POORLY DIFFERENTIATED THYROID CANCER

Anaplastic thyroid cancer (ATC) is a rare and aggressive cancer. It occurs in approximately 1 to 2 percent of thyroid cancer patients. While it is thought to be a variant form of papillary thyroid cancer, because it is undifferentiated, it is difficult to tell its origin. Since it is a rapidly growing cancer, once it has been determined that the cells are ATC, it needs to be treated quickly. Based on its aggressive behavior, ATC is classified as being Stage IV upon identification. Initially, ATC is harder to detect since it can grow unnoticed until a lump in the neck is observed or some hoarseness in the voice is heard. It may also be present with other types of thyroid cancers.

There is another cancer cell called poorly differentiated thyroid carcinoma (PDTC) which looks like and behaves in a similar manner as anaplastic thyroid cancer. It too is aggressive and, as its name indicates, poorly differentiated. While it is difficult to identify PDTC from ATC in its early stages, as the tumor grows, they differ from each other in appearance and smell according to surgeons who have operated on these two forms of cancer. PDTC and ATC are normally treated in the same manner.

Potential Spread

Anaplastic thyroid cancer is likely to spread to nearby lymph nodes. As it increases in size, it grows towards the larynx, trachea, and esophagus. It may commonly compress or invade the throat area resulting in hoarseness or respiratory difficulty. When it is discovered later in its development, it commonly spreads to the lungs and/or bones.

Tests

Ultrasound, scans, and/or a fine needle aspiration (FNA) may be performed. Because ATC is so rare, the initial FNA pathology results may be described as poorly differentiated cells, however, if it is not identified as ATC or of a cancerous nature, more tests should be done immediately.

Treatments

Because anaplastic thyroid cancer occurs so rarely, it is important to find a medical center that has had experience dealing with this form of cancer. (See Resources on page 183.)

Surgery. Surgery is normally first done to remove the tumor(s). This may require removal of one side of the thyroid gland or the complete thyroid based upon the tumor's involvement with the structures around it. Based upon how extensive the growth of the ATC is around the trachea, and esophagus, a tracheotomy may be performed to allow for easier breathing and a feeding tube inserted.

When there is extensive tumor growth around the structures in the neck, surgery may not be an option. In such cases, chemotherapy and/or external beam radiation may be used to shrink the tumor.

Radioactive iodine (RAI). Radioactive iodine (RAI) is not an option. Because ATC cells do not absorb iodine, RAI has little effect on this type of thyroid cancer.

External beam radiation therapy. After surgery, external beam radiation treatments are normally given. In some cases, a low dose of chemotherapy is included to enhance the effects of the radiation. The drug docetaxel, when used in conjunction with radiation, has shown some effectiveness.

Based on the length of this treatment, having a feeding tube inserted may be suggested.

Chemotherapy. Combination of chemotherapeutic agents may be an option, however such treatments have shown very limited effectiveness with one exception. ATC patients with the BRAF gene mutation shown positive results when given the combination of vemurafenib and dabrafenib.

Drugs. While there are a number of new targeted drugs available that are aimed at blocking the pathways necessary to the development and progression of the ATC cells, their effectiveness is limited. You can learn more about these drugs from your oncologist.

Clinical trials. There are a number of clinical trials available for ATC patients. (See Resources for more information on page 183.) Before entering any clinical trial, however, it is wise to ask what phase the trial is in, and what the preliminary results of the trials have shown.

Levothyroxine sodium. Once treatments have been completed, patients will normally be required to take the drug levothyroxine sodium, a synthetic thyroid hormone, for the rest of their lives.

Blood tests. Follow-up blood tests are normally given every 6 to 12 months to check on thyroid hormone levels.

Outcomes (Prognosis)

Patients who are able to identify this type of cancer early in its progression, with tumors that have little involvement around the structures in the neck, have a higher rate of survival. Unfortunately, in many cases, ATC becomes notable only after it has progressed to an advanced stage. Because of this, it is a difficult cancer to treat successfully.

OTHER CANCERS IN THE THYROID GLAND

The thyroid gland may also be the site of other types of cancers, such as the lung, kidney, and breast that have spread (metastasized) from other parts of the body. On the other hand, the thyroid may rarely be the site of metastasis from other primary tumors which include sarcomas, lymphomas, epidermoid carcinomas, and teratomas.

Hyperthyoidism and Cancer

Certain types of cancer cells can create an overproduction of thyroid hormones which can lead to hyperthyroidism, along with all of its signs and symptoms. (*See* page 163.) This can occur due to a pituitary tumor producing too much TSH or to thyroid cancer cells, capable of producing hormones, overproducing thyroid hormones. While these conditions are rare, it is important to be aware them. They include:

TSH-secreting Pituitary Adenomas

These are rare, slow growing pituitary tumors and account for about 1 to 2 percent of all pituitary adenomas that are removed through surgery. These tumors can be aggressive and invasive. They may also be a cause of hyperthyroidism.

Struma Ovarii

Struma ovarii is a rare tumor that occurs in a teratoma or dermoid of the ovary. It comprises about 1 percent of all ovarian tumors. It is often mixed with a carcinoid tumor and can occur in association with multiple endocrine neoplasia type IIA. The cause of struma ovarii is not known. Eight percent are benign and 90 percent are localized. Treatment is removal of the ovarian tumor. If the individual is thyrotoxic before surgery, then thionamides are given. B-adrenergic blocking medications may also need to be prescribed.

Thyrotoxicosis Caused By
Pregnancy and Trophoblastic Disease

Human chorionic gonadotropin (HCG) is a hormone that is produced in a pregnant woman. It has intrinsic TSH-like activity. In about 2 to 3 percent of normal pregnancies, gestational transient thyrotoxicosis is present due to elevated HCG concentrations. Familial gestational hyperthyroidism can also occur due to a gene mutation which makes the body hypersensitive to HCG. Thyrotoxicosis can also be induced by molar pregnancy and by trophoblastic disease in both men and women. In a molar pregnancy with hyperthyroidism, studies have shown that when the hydatidiform mole is removed, the thyrotoxicosis resolves.

**Thyrotoxicosis Caused By
Metastatic Differentiated Thyroid Carcinoma**

Thyrotoxicosis caused by functioning metastasis of differentiated thyroid carcinoma is uncommon. Eight-five percent of the people are over the age of 40 and it is more common in women than men. The clinical picture is the same for this disease as it is for other causes of thyrotoxicosis. Excessive thyroid hormone production is due to the large mass of metastatic tissue. Treatment is surgery or radioactive iodine.

Tests

Blood tests, ultrasound, scans, a fine needle aspiration (FNA), and/or personalized genetic test may be performed to determine the type of cancer it is.

Treatments

Once the specific type of cancer has been determined, the patient may be working with both an endocrinologist and oncologist specializing in the type of cancer found.

SUGGESTIONS

The stark reality is that over 60,000 people will be told that they have thyroid cancer this year—and sitting there, in a doctor's office, being told you have any type of cancer is not easy. The news tends to knock the wind right out of you. While the vast majority of thyroid cancer patients will be treated successfully, there are important things that a patient should consider doing in preparation for the journey that lies ahead of them. These same suggestions also hold true for those patients with more aggressive thyroid cancers. The better prepared you are, the better decisions you will be able to make.

Find the Right Advocate

An advocate is someone who will not only be with you as you go through the various stages of the process, but also ask questions and take notes when necessary. Most people, upon being told they have cancer, may hear the doctor talking, but they are in shock, and unable to respond appropriately, or remember what is being said. Therefore choosing the right advocate is important. Whether it's an adult child, spouse, parent, or friend, make sure that they have the time to be there with you, and that they will not be overwhelmed by the process.

If you don't have anyone that you can rely on, reach out to cancer support groups. They can be found online. They may be part of a nonprofit cancer group or they may be affiliated with a medical center. (See resources on page 183.) Many groups have volunteers that can be of assistance.

Learn as Much as You Can and Ask Questions

Making informed decisions is not always easy. The easiest path for some is to simply follow the instructions given by your doctor. Certainly there is nothing wrong with listening to what you doctor has to offer, however, you and/or your advocate should learn as much about the disease and your treatment options as possible. Too many people are afraid to ask questions.

There are a number of hard questions to ask such as: What are my chances of survival if I do this or do that? Are there any side effects from the treatments? Is there anything I can do to improve my odds? Have you treated this type of cancer before? When you don't understand something being told to you, tell them you don't understand, and ask them to explain it to you in simpler language. If you feel you are not satisfied with the information you are getting, do not hesitate to get second or third opinions from other health care professionals.

Be Prepared

It has been the Boy Scouts' motto for over one hundred years and there's a good reason why it should be yours. You need to be prepared for what lies in ahead of you. There are a number of important things to consider:

- Always take copies of all your test results with you on your visits to doctors or medical centers, especially if you are visiting them for the first time. If a past scan is available only in an electronic form, have the laboratory provide you with a copy on a CD. You will find that it is a standard practice for doctors to request laboratory reports be sent to them before your visit. However, many times you show up, but the reports have not. Be prepared!

- Learn as much as you can about any procedures that you will be undergoing. Whether it's a scan, an insertion of a feeding tube, an operation, the necessary preparation for radiation—learn what's involved. For example, some scans involve being put into a tubular enclosure. If this is a problem for you, ask if they have an open scanner, or perhaps ask for something to calm you down. Also, ask how long these procedures take. It's helpful to know since you now have to work your life around their schedules. Be prepared!

- Ask questions about any and all of the possible side effects of any procedure. Over the years, many drugs have been developed to either overcome or lessen side effects. There may also be natural remedies that might help alleviate some of these problems. Know what remedies are out there ahead of time. Be prepared!

- Take things to do with you while you wait. Read a book, take an iPad, listen to music, do a crossword puzzle, text a friend—take something along that can help pass the time. As you will discover, there is a reason they are called waiting rooms, so be prepared!

- Consider joining a thyroid cancer listserv. The term listserv refers to on-line groups devoted to working with thyroid cancer patients and their advocates. These groups are normally composed of current patients, survivors, advocates, and in some cases, medical professionals who can answer your questions about almost anything related to your situation. They can provide information based upon their own experiences. They can likewise be a source of great support in understanding that you are not alone. (See Resources, page 183.) Be prepared!

It is not uncommon for you to feel as though you are not in control of your present circumstances. The suggestions above should help to empower you as a patient. By preparing in advance—by knowing what to ask and what to do—you will find that you do have some control over the process.

CONCLUSION

I have heard it said that if you are going to get cancer, thyroid cancer is the best one to get. Personally, I don't think any cancer fits that description. What I will say is that modern medicine has been able to treat the vast majority of thyroid cancers successfully. Additionally, some of the new genetic tests allow patients to learn relatively quickly whether a node is benign or malignant. However, there are enough rare and aggressive forms of these cancers to make the journey that much more difficult. If there is one key to beating thyroid cancer, it is to find it early, take immediate action, and to consider the spiritual component of your life. Therefore, make sure your tests and treatments don't rely on someone else's timetable. I hope the information in this chapter equips you with the appropriate questions in making the decisions that are right for you.

Conclusion

Hopefully by now, you have come to understand the critical role that the thyroid gland and its hormones play in your ability to think, to feel, and to sustain the many systems that keep you alive and functioning normally. As you have seen in the chapters of this book, when the thyroid gland does not function correctly, it can cause any number of serious problems. Too often, the underlying cause of these difficulties goes undetected.

The purpose of my writing this book has been to provide you with a clear understanding of how the thyroid gland works and what thyroid hormones do to keep the body functioning optimally. Literally tens of thousands of men and women suffer from a wide variety of thyroid-related health issues and are unaware of the source of their symptoms and signs. Because their condition may be subclinical—in other words, it may not be detected by physical examinations or standard blood tests—patients are sometimes prescribed drugs that are not thyroid hormones to diminish their overt symptoms. Add to that the fact that the number of people with thyroid problems is rapidly growing, and you can see the difficulty that lies ahead for so many individuals.

If you or a loved one suffers from some of the symptoms described in this book, and you have not been able to isolate their cause, I hope you consider acting as an advocate and asking your healthcare provider to determine if these ailments are thyroid-related. If, on the other hand, you have been diagnosed with a thyroid issue that is covered in this book, I hope I have been able to provide you with a clearer understanding of what the problem is and how it can be treated. Knowledge is power, and your ability to ask the right questions and understand the answers will, in turn, enable you to make informed decisions about your health.

Always be aware that medicine is a rapidly changing science, and that while I have done my best to provide you with up-to-date information, new tests and treatments are always emerging. View this book as a springboard to further investigation, and be certain that you have all the available facts before making a decision regarding treatment. As long as you understand that you have a significant role to play in overcoming your thyroid disorder, you will have taken an important step toward greater health.

Resources

NATURAL MEDICINE SPECIALISTS

To ensure optimal health, it is important to work with a healthcare practitioner who will be take your medical history into account in formulating a personal regimen for you. Below, you'll find a list of organizations that can lead you to local professionals who specialize in Functional Medicine, Anti-Aging Medicine, and Personalized Medicine.

American Academy of Anti-Aging Physicians
1801 North Military Trail, Suite 200
Boca Raton, FL 33431
(888) 997-0112
www.a4m.com

Institute for Functional Medicine
505 Soth 336th Street, Suite 500
Federal Way, WA 98003
(800) 228-0622
(253) 661-3010
www.functionalmedicine.org

DIAGNOSTIC LABORATORIES

The following is a list of diagnostic laboratories that offer tests to evaluate your genetics, hormone and nutrient levels, gastrointestinal function, and heavy metal exposure. These tests can be instrumental in identifying whether you are genetically predisposed to cognitive decline heart disease, or whether heavy metal poisoning, hormonal imbalance, nutritional deficiency, or inflammation is affecting your memory. Before ordering any medical test, consult with your healthcare practitioner.

Doctor's Data Laboratory
3755 Illinois Avenue
St. Charles, IL 60174
(800) 323-2784
www.doctorsdata.com

Genova Diagnostic Laboratory/ Metametrix Clinical Laboratory
63 Zillicoa Street
Asheville, NC 28801
(800) 522-4762
www.gdx.net

Neuroscience Laboratory
373 280th Street
Osceloa, WI 54020

Pathways Genomics Corporation
4045 Sorrento Valley Blvd.
San Diego CA, 92121
(877) 505-7374
www.pathway.com

Spectracell Laboratories
10401 Town Park Drive
Houston, Texas 77072
(800) 227-5227
(713) 621-3101
www.spectracell.com

ZRT Laboratory
8605 Southwest Creekside Place
Beaverton, OR 97006
(866) 600-1635
www.zrtlab.com

CANCER

American Thyroid Association
The American Thyroid Association is devoted to thyroid biology and to the prevention and treatment of thyroid disease through research, clinical care, education, and public health. It covers scientific inquiry, clinical excellence, public service, patient advocacy, and education.

American Thyroid Association
6066 Leesburg Pike, Suite 550
Falls Church, Virginia 22041
phone: (703) 998-8890 • fax: (703) 998-8893
General website: www.thyroid.org
e-mail: thyroid@thyroid.org

National Cancer Institute (NCI)
National Cancer Institute provides information on all types of cancers including thyroid cancer on their site. In addition to explaining what these cancers are and how they are normally treated, it offers a listing of clinical trials taking place throughout the country.

National Institutes of Health
Bethesda, MD 20892
General website: www.cancer.gov
Thyroid Cancer related: www.cancer.gov/types/thyroid
Clinical Trials: www.cancer.gov/about-cancer/treatment/clinical-trials/search

ThyCa: Thyroid Cancer Survivors' Association, Inc.
This non-profit organization provides information to education patients and their families about all types and aspects of thyroid cancer including clinical trial information, medical specialists, and the contacts for other thyroid cancer-related organizations.

In addition, ThyCa offers online community support groups in which patients, family members, advocates, and survivors can communicate with each other on a one-on-one setting or within a group. ThyCA support groups include Advanced Thyroid Cancer Support Group, Anaplastic Support Group, Caregivers Support Group, Childbearing and Thyroid Cancer Group, Long-Term Survivors Support Group, Love, Loss, & Legacy Group, Medullary Support Groups, Pediatric Support Group, Thyca—Thyroid Cancer Support Group (mainly papillary and follicular) , ThyCa Mental Challenges Support Group, ThyCa Young Adults Support Group, Monday Evening Online Chat Room for Thyroid Cancer Survivors, and Groups Not Affiliated with ThyCa.

ThyCA
PO Box 1545
New York, NY 10159-1545
Phone: (877) 588-7904 (Toll-Free) • Fax: (630) 604-6078
General website: www.thyca.org
ThyCa Support Groups: www.thyca.org/sg/email/

"FDA Approves Zelboraf (Vemurafenib) and Companion Diagnostic for BRAF Mutation-Positive Metastatic Melanoma, a Deadly Form of Skin Cancer" (Press release). Genentech. Retrieved 2011-08-17.

DEPRESSION

From *Harvard Mental Health Letter:* This issue covers the treatment of an underactive thyroid which may improve one's mood. It explains why there is a link between hypothyroidism and depression.
www.health.harvard.edu/newsletter_article/when-depression-starts-in-the-neck

From the *New York Times:* Research exploring a link between thyroid problems (minor or subclinical) and psychiatric difficulties.
www.nytimes.com/2011/11/22/health/for-some-psychiatric-troubles-may-begin-with-the-thyroid.html?_r=0

CELIAC DISEASE

Celiac disease is an autoimmune disorder that can occur in genetically pre-disposed people where the ingestion of gluten leads to damage in the small intestine. The Celiac Disease Foundation supports advancing research to improve the quality of life for those affected by gluten-free disorders.

Celiac Disease Foundation
20350 Ventura Blvd Ste 240
Woodland Hills, CA 91364
Phone: (818) 716-1513
Fax: (818) 267-5577

GUT BACTERIA

H. Pylori
From Healthline: Explores the issue of a thyroid and acid reflux (GERD) connection. www.healthline.com/health/gerd/thyroid

PERSONALIZED GENETIC TESTING

From University of Pittsburgh Cancer Institute: Newly available testing that incorporates personalized medicine into diagnosing the thyroid cancer condition.
http://globenewswire.com/news-release/2015/07/06/750020/10140729/en/Pitt-Scientists-Lead-Consensus-Guidelines-for-Thyroid-Cancer-Molecular-Tests.html

References

INTRODUCTION

Hollenberg, A., and Jameson, J., Mechanism of Thyroid Hormone Action. In Degroot, L, and Jameson, J., Endocrinology. 5th Ed. Vol 2, p. 1873–97.

CHAPTER 1. YOU AND YOUR THYROID

Ames, B., et al., "Oxidants, antioxidants, and the degenerative diseases of aging," *Proc Natl Acad Sci SA* 1993; 90(17):7915–22.

Bengtsson, A., et al., "Reduced high-energy phosphate levels in the painful muscles of patients with primary fibromyalgia," *Arthritis and Rheumatism* 1986: 29(7):817–21.

Bengtsson, A., et al., "The muscle in fibromyalgia: a review of Swedish studies," *Jour of Rheumatology* 1989: 16(Suppl 19):144–49.

Brehm, A., et al., "Increased lipid availability impairs insulin-stimulated ATP synthesis in human skeletal muscle," *Diabetes* 2006; 55:136–40.

Burroughs, S. et al., "Depression and anxiety. Role of mitochondria," *Current Anesthesia Crit Care* 2007; 18:34–41.

Chen, L., et al., "Depressed mitochondrial fusion in heart failure," *Circulation* 2007; 116:259.

Corral-Debrinski, M., et al., "Association of mitochondrial DNA damage with aging and coronary atherosclerotic heart disease," *Mutat Res* 1992; 275(3–6):169–80.

Daimon, C., et al., "The role of thyrotropin releasing hormone in aging and neurodegenerative diseases," *Amer Jour Alz Dis (Columbia)* 2013; 1(1) .

De Jong, M., et al., "Transport of 3,5,3' triiodothyronine into the perfused rat liver subsequent metabolism are inhibited by fasting," *Endocrinology* 1992; 131(1):463–70.

Demarco, N., et al., "Effect of fasting on free fatty acid, glycerol and cholesterol concentrations in blood plasma and lipoprotein lipase activity in adipose tissue of cattle," *Jour Anim Sci* 1981; 52:75–82.

Elliot, D., et al., "Sustained depression of the resting metabolic rate after massive weight loss," *Amer Jour Clin Nutr* 1989; 49:93–6.

Everts, M., et al., "Effects of a furan fatty acid and indoxyl sulfate on thyroid hormone uptake in cultured anterior pituitary cells," *Amer Jour Physiol* 1995; 268:E974-E979.

Fattal, O., et al., "Review of the literature on major mental disorders in adults patients with mitochondrial diseases," *Psychosomatics* 2006; 47(1):1–7.

Fullle, S., et al., "Specific oxidative alterations in vastus lateralls muscle of patients with the diagnosis of chronic fatigue syndrome," *Free Radic Biol Med* 2000; 29(12):1252–59.

Gardner, A., et al., "Mitochondrial energy depletion in depression with somatization," *Psychother Psychosom* 2006; 77:17–29.

Goglia, F., "Biological effects of 3–5-diiodothyronine, T2," *Biochemistry (Mosc)* 2005; 70 (2):164–72.

Henemann, G. Hennemann, G., et al., "Plasma membrane transport of thyroid hormones and its role in thyroid hormone metabolism and bioavailability," Endocrine Rev 2001; 22(4):451–76.

Hennemann, G., et al., "Decreased peripheral 3,5,3'-triiodothyroxine (T3) production from thyroxine (T4) . A syndrome of impaired thyroid hormone activation due to transport inhibition of T4-into T3-producing tissues," *Jour Cliln Endocrinol Metabol* 1993; 77(5):1431–35.

Hennemann, G., et al., "The kinetics of thyroid hormone transporters and their role in nonthyroidal illness and starvation," *Best Practice and Res Clin Endoc Metabol* 2007; 21(2):323–38.

Hollenberg, A., and Jameson, J., Mechanism of Thyroid Hormone Action. In Degroot, L, and Jameson, J., Endocrinology. 5th Ed. Vol 2, p. 1873–97.

Holm, A., et al., "Kinetics of triiodothyronine uptake by erythrocytes in hyperthyroidism, hypotroidism, and thyroid hormone resistance," *Jour Clin Endocrinol Metab* 1989; 69:364–68.

Hutchin, T., et al., "A mitochondrial DNA clone is associat3ed with increased risk for Alzheimer's disease," *Proc Nat Acad Sci USA* 1995; 92:6892–96.

Kamath, J., et al., "The thyrotropin-releasing hormone (TRH) immune system homeostatic hypothesis," *Pharm Ther* 2009; 121(1):20–8.

Kaptein, E., "Clinical relevance of thyroid hormone alterations in nonthyroidal illness," *Thyroid Int* 1997; 4:22–5.

Kaptein, E., "Thyroid hormone metabolism and thyroid disease in chronic renal failure," *Endocr Rev* 1996; 17:45–63.

Kaptein, E., et al., "Peripheral serum thyroxine, triiodothyronine in the low thyroxine state of acute nonthyroidal illness. A noncompartmental analysis," *Jour Clin Invest* 1982; 69:526–35.

Krenning, E., et al., "Characteristics of active transport of thyroid hormone into rat hepatocytes," *Biochim Biophys Acta* 1981; 676:14–20.

Leibel, R., et al., "Diminished energy requirements in reduced-obese patients," *Metabolism* 1984; 33(2):164–70.

Miquel, J., et al., "Mitochondrial role in cell aging," *Exp Gerontol* 1980; 15:575–91.

Papa, S., "Mitochondrial phosphorylation changes in the life span. Molecular aspects and physiopathological implications," *Biochimica Biophysica Acta* 1996; 87–105.

Park, J., et al., "Evidence for metabolic abnormalities in the muscles of patients with fibromyalgia," *Curr Rheumatool Rep* 2000; 2(2):131–40.

Petersen, K., et al., "Decreased insulin-stimulated ATP synthesis and phosphate transport in muscle of insulin-resistance offspring of type 2 diabetic patients," *PLoS Med* 2005; 2(9):e233.

Pieczenik, S., et al., "Mitochondrial dysfunction and molecular pathways of disease," *Exp Mol Pathol* 2007; 83(1):84–92.

Puddu, P., et al., "Mitochondrial dysfunction as an initiating event in atherogenesis: a plausible hypothesis," *Cardiology* 2005; 103(3):137–41.

Richter, C., "Oxidative damage to mitochondrial DNA and its relationship to aging," *Int Jour Biochem Cell Biol* 1995; 27(7):647–53.

Riley, W., et al., "Characterization of 3,5,3'triiodo-thyroxine transport into hepatocytes isolated from juvenile rainbow trout (Oncorhynchus mykiss), and comparison with L-thyroxine transport," *Gen Comp Endocrinol* 1994; 95:301–09.

Savitha, S., et al., "Efficacy of levo carnitine and alpha lipoic acid in ameliorating the decline in mitochondrial enzymes during aging," *Clin Nutr* 2005; 24(5):794–800.

Schapria, A., "Mitochondrial disease," Lancet 2006; 368:70–82.

Sherer, T., et al., "Environment, mitochondria, and Parkinson's disease," *Neuroscientist* 2002; 8(3):192–97.

Spenser, C., et al., "Dynamics of serum thyrotropin and thyroid hormone changes in fasting," *Jour Clin Endocrin Metab* 1983; 5:883–88.

Stavrovskaya, I., et al., "The powerhouse takes control of the cell: is the mitochondrial permeability transition a viable therapeutic target against neuronal dysfunction and death?" *Free Radic Biol Med* 2005; 38(6):687–97.

Stork, C., et al., "Mitochondrial dysfunction in bipolar disorder: evidence from magnetic resonance spectroscopy research," *Mol Psychiatry* 2005; 10(10):900–19.

Szendroedi, J., et al., "Impaired mitochondrial function and insulin resistance of skeletal muscle in mitochondrial diabetes," *Diabetes Care* 2009; 32(4):677–79.

Verga, S., et al., "A low reported energy intake is associated with metabolic syndrome," *Jour Endocrinol Invest* 2009; 32:538–41.

West, I., "Radicals and oxidative stress in diabetes," *Diabet Med* 2000; 17(3):171–80.

CHAPTER 2. HYPOTHYROIDISM

Abraham, G., et al., "The safe and effective implementation of orthoiodosupplementation in medical practice," *The Original Internist*, April 2004.

Adlin, V., et al., "Subclinical hypothyroidism: deciding when to treat," *Amer Fam Physician* 1998; 57(4):776–80.

Althaus, U., et al., "LDL/HDL-changes in subclinical hypothyroidism: possible risk factors for coronary heart disease," *Clin Endocrinol* 19898; 28:157–63.

Anker, G. et al., "Thyroid function in post-menopausal breast cancer patients treated with Tamoxifen," *Scandinavian Jour of Clin Labor Invest* 1998; 58:103–07.

Arnold, L., "Alternative treatments for adults with attention-deficit hyperactivity disorder (ADHD) ," *Ann NY Acad Sci* 2001; 931:310–41.

Berger, N., et al., "Influence of selenium supplementation on the post-traumatic alterations of the thyroid axis: a placebo-controlled trial," *Intensive Care Med* 2001; 27(1):91–100.

Berry, M., et al., "The role of selenium in thyroid hormone action," *Endocrine Rev* 1992; 13:207–20.

Biondi, B., et al., "Combination treatment with T4 and T3: toward personalized replacement therapy in hypothyroidism," *Jour Clin Endocrinol Metab* 2012; 97(7):2256–71.

Brownstein, D., Iodine: *Why You Need It, Why You Can't Live Without It*. Medical Alternatives Press, 2004.

Brucker-David, F., "Effects of environmental synthetic chemicals on thyroid function," *Thyroid* 1998; 8(9):827–56.

Bunevicious, R.,, et al., "Effect of thyroxine as compared with thyroxine plus triiodothyronine in patients with hypothyroidism," *NEJM* 1994; 340(6):424–29.

Campbell, N., et al., "Ferrous sulfate reduces thyroxine efficacy in patients with hypothyroidism," *Ann Intern Med* 1992; 117(12):1010–13.

Cappola, A., et al., "Hypothyroidism and atherosclerosis," *Jour Clin Endocrinol Metab* 2003; 88:2438–44.

Cavalieri, R., et al., Effects of drugs on human thyroid hormone metabolism. In Hennemann G (ed): Thyroid Hormone Metabolism. New York: Marcel Dekker, 1998; p. 359–79.

Christianson, A., and Murray, M., Hypothyroidism. In Pizzorno, J., and Murray, M., Textbook of Natural Medicine. St. Louis: Elsevier/Churchill Livingstone, 2013, p. 1473–80.

Contempre, B., et al. "Effect of selenium supplementation on thyroid hormone metabolism in an iodine and selenium deficient population," *Clin Endocrinol* 1992; 36:579–83.

Dean, J., et al., "Exaggerated responsiveness to thyrotrophin releasing hormone: a risk factor in women with artery disease," *Brit Med Jour (Clin Res Ed)* 1985; 290:1555–61.

DeGroot, L., *Endocrinology*. 5th edition. Philadelphia: Elsevier Saunders, 2006.

Deyssig, R., et al., "Ingestion of androgenic-anabolic steroids induces mild thyroidal impairment in male body builders," *Jour Clin Endocrinol Metab* 1993; 76(4):1069–71.

Divi, R., et al., "Anti-thyroid isoflavones from soybean: isolation, characterization, and mechanism of action," *Biochem Pharmacol* 1997; 54(10):1087–96.

Duick, D., et al., "Effect of single dose dexamethasone on the concentration of serum triiodothyronine in man," *Jour Clin Endocrin Metab* 1974; 39(6):1151–54.

Evans, T., "Thyroid disease," *Prim Care* 2003; 30:625–40.

Feidt-Rasmussen, U., et al., "Effect of clomifene on thyroid function in normal men," *Acta Endocrinol* 1979; 90(1):43–51.

Fernandez-Real, J., et al., "Thyroid function is intrinsically linked to insulin sensitivity and endothelium—dependent vasodilation in healthy euthyroid subjects," *Jour Clin Endocrin Met* 2006; June 27.

Glinoer, D., et al., "Use of direct thyroxine-binding globulin measurement in the evaluation of thyroid function," *Jour Endocrinol Invest* 1978; 1(4):329–35.

Gold, M., et al., "Hypothyroidism and depression, evidence from complete thyroid function evaluation," *JAMA* 1981; 245:1919–22.

Hertoghe, J., et al., "Thyroid insufficiency. Is thyroxine the only valuable drug?" *Jour of Nutr & Environ Med* 2001; 11:159–66.

Hochberg, M., et a., "Hypothyroidism presenting as a polymyositis-like syndrome," *Arthr Rheum* 1976; 19:1363–66.

Hollowell, J., et al., *Jour of Clin Endo Met* 2002; 87(2):489–99.

Huseman, C., et al, "Childhood lead toxicity and impaired release of thyroid stimulation hormone," *Environ Res* 1987; 42:524–33.

Jakobs, T., et al., "Proinflammatory cytokines inhibit the expression and function of human type I 5'deiodinase in HepG2 hepatocarcinoma cells," *Eur Jour Endo* 2002; 146(4):559–66.

Jorgensen, J., et al., "Effects of growth hormone on thyroid function of growth hormone-deficient adults with and without concomitant thyroxine-substituted central hypothyroidism," *Jour Clin Endocrinol Metab* 1989; 69(6):1127–32.

Kidd, P., et al., "ADHD in children: rationale for its integrative management," *Alt Med Rev* 2000; 5(5):402–28.

Kirkegaard, C., et al., "Studies on the influence of biogenic amines and psychoactive drugs on the prognostic value of TRH stimulation test in endogenous depression," *Psychoneuroendocrinology* 1977; 2(2):131–36.

Kirkegaard, C., et al., "Thyrotrophin-releasing hormone (TRH) stimulation test in manic depressive illness," *Arch Gen Pschiatr* 1978; 35(8):1017–21.

Kohrle, J., "The deiodinase family, selenoenzymes regulating thyroid hormone availability and action," *Cell Mol Life Sci* 2000; 57:1853–63.

Krupsky, M., et al., "Musculoskeletal symptoms as a presenting sign of long-standing hypothyroidism," *Isr Jour Med Sci* 1987; 23:1110–13.

Lange, U., et al., Thyroid disorders in female patients with ankylosing spondylitis," *Eur Jour Med Res* 1999; 4(11):468–74.

Lazarus, J., et al., "Lithium therapy and thyroid function: A long-term study," *Psychol Med* 1981; 11(1):85–92.

Leung, A., et al., "Iodine-induced thyroid dysfunction," Current Opinion in Endocrinology, Diabetes, and Obesity 2012; 19(5):414–19.

Leznoff, A., et, al., "Syndrome of idiopathic chronic urticaria and angioedema with thyroid autoimmuity: a study of 90 patients," *Jour of Allergy and Clinical Immunology* 1989; 84(1):66–71.

McCowen, K., et al., "Elevated serum thyrotropin in thyroxine-treated patients with hypothyroidism given sertraline," NEJM 1997; 337(14):1010-11.

Meinhold, H., et al., "Effects of selenium and iodine deficiency on iodothyronine deiodinases in brain, thyroid and peripheral tissue," *JAMA* 1992; 19:8–12.

Neeck, G., et al., "Neuroendocrine perturbations in fibromyalgia and chronic fatigue syndrome," *Rheum Dis Clin North Amer* 2000; 26(4):989–1002.

Nelis, G., et al., "The effect of oral cimetidine on the basal and stimulated values of prolactin, thyroid stimulating hormone, follicle stimulating hormone and luteinizing hormone," *Postgrad Med Jour* 1980; 56(651):26–9.

Newman, C., et al., "Amiodarone and the thyroid: A practical guide to the management of thyroid dysfunction induced by amiodarone therapy," *Heart* 1998; 79:121–27.

Nishida, M., et al., "Direct evidence for the presence of methylmercury bound in the thyroid and other organs obtained from mice given methylmercury; differentiation of free and bound methylmercuries in biological materials determined by volatility of methylmercury," *Chem Pharm Bull* 1990; 38(5):1412–13.

Nishiyama, S. et al., "Zinc supplementation alters thyroid hormone metabolism in disabled patients with zinc deficiency," *Jour Amer Coll Nutr* 1994; 13:62–7.

Northcutt, R., et al., "The influence of cholestyramine on thyroxine absorption," *JAMA* 1969; 208(10):1857–61.

Pansini, F., "Effect of the hormonal contraception on serum reverse triiodothyronine levels," *Gynecol Obstet Invest* 1987; 23:133.

Portes, E., et al., "Changes in serum thyroid hormones levels and their mechanisms during long-term growth hormone (GH) replacement therapy in GH deficient children," *Clin Endocrinol* 2000; 53(2):183–89.

Propranolol and thyroid hormone metabolism," *Thyroid* 1991; 1:273–77.

Rachman, B., "Managing endocrine imbalance; autoimmune-induced thyroidopathy and chronic fatigue syndrome," Functional Medicine Approaches to Endocrine Disturbances of aging. Gig Harbor Washington: The Institute For Functional Medicine, 2001; p. 226.

Rootwelt, K., et al., "Effect of carbamazepine, phenytoin and phenobarbital on serum levels of thyroid hormones and thyrotropin in humans," *Scand Jour Clin Lab Invest* 1978; 38(8):731–36.

Rose, N., et al., "The role of iodine in autoimmune thyroiditis," *Clin Reviews in Immunology* 1997; 17:511–17.

Rouzier, N., "Thyroid replacement therapy," Longevity and Preventive Medicine Symposium, 2002; p. 2.

Schlienger, J., et al., "The action of clomipramine on thyroid function," *Horm Metab Res* 1980; 12(9):481–82.

Sherman, S., et al., "Sucralfate causes malabsorption of L-thyroxine," *Amer Jour Med* 1994; 96(6):531–35.

Shomon, M., *Living Well With Hypothyroidism*. New York: Avon Books, Inc., 2000.

Singh N., et al., "Effect of calcium carbonate on the absorption of levothyroxine," *JAMA* 2000; 283(21):2822–25.

Smith, J., et al., "Thyroid hormones, brain function and cognition: a brief review," *Neurosci Biobehav Rev* 2002; 26:45–60.

Smith, P., *What You Must Know About Women's Hormones*. Garden City Park, NY: Square One Publishing, 2010.

Sperber, A., et al., "Evidence for interference with the intestinal absorption of levothyroxine sodium by aluminum hydroxide," *Arch Intern Med* 1992; 152(1):183–84.

St. Germain, D., "Selenium, deiodinases, and endocrine function", In Hatfield (ed): Selenium Its Molecular Biology and Role in Human Health. Boston: Kluwer, 2001, p. 189–202.

Starr, M., Hypothyroidism: Type 2. Columbia, MO: Mark Starr Trust, 2005.

Takasu, N., et al., "Rifampin-induced hypothyroidism in patients with Hashimoto's thyroiditis," *NEJM* 2005; 352(5):518–19.

Torpy, D., et al., "Acute and delayed effects of a single-dose injection of interleukin-6 on thyroid function in healthy humans," *Metabolism* 1998; 47(10):1289–93.

Tseng, A., et al., "Interaction between ritonavir and levothyroxine," AIDS 1998; 12(16):2235–36.

Turnbridge, W., et al., "Lipid profiles and cardiovascular disease in the Wickham area with particular reference to thyroid failure," *Clin Endocrinol* 1977; 7:495–508.

Wartofsky, L., "Combination L-T3 and L-T4 therapy for hypothyroidism," Curr Opin Endocrinology Diabetes Obes 1013; 20(5):460–66.

Wartofsky, L., et al., "The evidence for a narrower thyrotropin reference range is compelling," *Jour Clin Endo Met* 2005; 90(9):5483–88.

WHO, November 12, 1998.

Woeber, K., "Levothyroxine therapy and serum free thyroxine and free triiodothyronine concentrations," *Jour Endocrinol Invest* 2002; 25(2):106–09.

CHAPTER 3. HYPERTHYROIDISM

Abe, E., et al., "TSH is a negative regulator of skeletal remodeling," *Cell* 2003; 115:151–62.

Aliciguzel, Y., et al., "Erythrocyte, plasma, and serum antioxidant activities in untreated toxic multinodular goiter patients," *Free Rad Biol Med* 2001; 15; 30:665–70.

Amino, N., *Postpartum Thyroid Disease*. In Bercu, B ., Shulman D., (Eds.) Advances in Perinatal Thyroidology. New York: Plenum, 1991, p. 167.

Aufmkolk, M., et al., "Antihormonal effects of plant extracts. Iodothyronine deiodinase of rat liver is inhibited by extracts and secondary metabolites of plants," *Horm Met Res* 1984; 16:188–92.

Aufmkolk, M., et al., "Inhibition by certain plant extracts of the binding and adenylate cyclase stimulatory effects of bovine thyrotropin in human thyroid membranes," *Endocrinology* 1984; 115:527–34.

Aufmkolk, M., et al., "The active principals of plant extracts with antithyroid activity: oxidation products of derivatives of 3,4-diihydrooxycinnamic acid," *Endocrinology* 1985; 116:1677–86.

Barbesino, G., et al., "Linkage analysis of candidate genes in autoimmune thyroid disease: II. Selected gender-related genes and the X-chromosome. International Consortium for the Genetics of Autoimmune Thyroid Disease," *Jour Clin Endocrinol Metabol* 1998; 83:3290–95.

Bartalena, I., et al., "Cigarette smoking and the thyroid," *Eur Jour Endocrinol* 1995; 133: 507–12.

Bartalena, L., et al., "Adverse effects of thyroid hormone preparations and antithyroid drugs," *Drug Saf* 1996; 15:53–63.

Barzilai, D., et al., "Fatal complications following use of potassium perchlorate in thyrotoxicosis. Report of two cases and a review of the literature," 1st *Jour Med Sci* 1966; 2:453–56.

Bassett, J., et al., "The molecular actions of thyroid hormone in bone," *Trends Endocrinol Metab* 2003; 14:356–64.

Beirerwaltes, W., "Treatment of hyperthyroidism with I-131. in Falk, S., (Ed.) Thyroid Disease: Endocrinology, Surgery, Nuclear Medicine and Radiotherapy. New York: Raven Press, 1990; p 233.

Benson, R., et al., "The menstrual pattern in hyperthyroidism and subsequent post therapy hypothyroidism," *Surg Gynecol Obstet* 1955; 100(1):19–26.

Benvenga, S., et al., "Usefulness of L-carnitine, a naturally occurring peripheral antagonist of thyroid hormone action in iatrogenic hyperthyroidism: a randomized, double-blind, placebo-controlled clinical trial," *Jour Clin Endocrinol Metab* 2001; 86:3579–94.

Blumenthal, M., et al., The Complete German Commission E Monographs: Therapeutic Guide to Herbal Medicine. Boston: American Botanical Council, 1998.

Bove, M., et al., Endocrine Disorders and Adrenal Support. In Romm, A., Botanical Medicine for Women's Health. St. Louis: Churchill Livingstone/Elsevier, 2010, p. 193–97.

Bransom, C., et al., "Solitary toxic adenoma of the thyroid gland," Brit Jour Surg 1997; 66:590.

Brauman, A., et al., "Prevalence of mitral valve prolapse in chronic lymphocytic thyroiditis and nongoitrous hypothyroidism," *Cardiology* 1988; 75:269–73.

Brent, G., et al., Hypothyroidism and Thyroiditis. In Melmed, S., et al. (Eds.) Williams Textbook of Endocrinology 12th Ed. Philadelphia: Saunders/Elsevier, 2011, 433–39.

Brownlie, B., et al., "Psychoses associated with thyrotoxicosis—thyrotoxic psychosis. A report of 18 cases with statistical analysis of incidence," *Eur Jour Endocrinol* 2000; 142(5):702–44.

Burggraaf, J., et al., "Sympathovagal imbalance in hyperthyroidism" *Amer Jour Physiol Endocrinol Metabol* 2001; 281:E190–95.

Burgi, H., et al., "Changes of circulating thyroxine, triiodothyronine and reverse triiodothyronine after radiographic contrast agents," *Jour Clin Endocrinol Metabol* 1976; 43:1203–10.

Cappola, A., et al., "Thyroid status, cardiovascular risk, and mortality in older adults," *JAMA* 2006; 295:1033–41.

Carani, C., et al., "Multicenter study on the prevalence of sexual symptoms in male hypo- and hyperthyroid patients," *Jour Clin Endocrinol Metab* 2005; 90(12):6472–79.

Carvalho-Bianco, S., et al., "Chronic cardiac-specific thyrotoxicosis increases myocardial beta-adrenergic responsiveness," *Mol Endocrinol* 2004; 18:1840–49.

Chang, D., et al., "The effect of preoperative Lugol's iodine on thyroid blood flow in patients with hyperthyroidism," *Surgery* 1987; 102:1055–61.

Chiovato, L., et al., "Disappearance of humoral thyroid autoimmunity after complete removal of thyroid antigens," *Ann Internal Med* 2003; 139:346–51.

Cooper, D., "Hyperthyroidism," *Lancet* 2003; 362(9382) 459–68.

Coulombe, P., et al., "Plasma catecholamine concentrations in hyperthyroidism and hypothyroidism," *Metabolism* 1976; 25:973–79.

Davis, P., "Hyperthyroidism in patients over the age of 60 years: clinical features in 85 patients," *Medicine (Baltimore)* 1974:53:161–81.

DeGroot, I., et al., "Effect of perchlorate and methimazole on iodine metabolism," *Acta Endocrinol (Copenh)* 1971; 68:696–706.

Dobyns, B., et al., "Functional and histologic effects of therapeutic doses of radioiodine therapy for hyperthyroidism," *Jour Clin Endocrinol Metabol* 1953; 13:548.

Doniach, D., "Humoral and genetic aspects of thyroid autoimmunity," *Clin Endocrinol Metabol* 1975; 4:267–68.

Emerson, C., et al., "Serum thyroxine and triiodothyronine concentrations during iodide treatment of hyperthyroidism," *Jour Clin Endocrinol Metabol* 1975; 40:33–6.

Emrich, D., et al., "Determination of the automatously functioning volume of the thyroid," *Eur Jour Nucl Med* 1993; 20:410.

Erem, C., et al., "Blood coagulation and fibrinolysis in patients with hyperthyroidism," *Jour Endocrinol Invest* 2002; 25:345–50.

Fazio, S., et al., "Effects of thyroid hormone on the cardiovascular system," *Recent Prog Horm Res* 2004; 59:31–50.

Galofre, J., et al., "Increased incidence of thyrotoxicosis after iodine supplementation in an iodine sufficient area," *Jour Endocrinol Invest* 1994; 17:23–7.

Gartner, R., et al., "Selenium supplementation in patients with autoimmune thyroiditis decreases thyroid peroxidase antibodies concentrations," *Jour Clin Endocrinol Metabol* 2002; 87(4):1687–91.

Ghosh, N., et al., "Thyrotoxicosis of the chlorides of cadmium and mercury in rabbit," *Biomed Environ Sci* 1992; 5:236–40.

Guimaraes, V., Subacute and Riedel's Thyroiditis. In DeGroot, L., Jameson, J., (Eds) . Endocrinology 5th Ed. Philadelphia: Saunders/Elsevier, 2006, p. 2069–80.

Gurlek, A., et al., "Liver tests in hyperthyroidism: effect of antithyroid therapy," Jour Clin Gastroenterol 1997; 24:180–83.

Hamburger, J., "Evolution of toxicity in solitary non-functioning thyroid nodules," *Jour Clin Endocrinol Metab* 1980; 50:1089.

Hawkes, W., et al., "Dietary selenium intake modulates thyroid hormone and energy metabolism in men," *Jour Nutr* 2003; 133:3443–48.

Hegedus, L., et al., Multinodular Goiter. In DeGroot, L., Jameson, J., (Eds) . Endocrinology 5th Ed. Philadelphia: Saunders/Elsevier, 2006, p. 2113–27.

Hellstrom, L., et al., "Catecholamine-induced adipocyte lipolysis in human hyperthyroidism," *Jour Clin Endocrinol Metabol* 1997; 82:159–66,

Henderson, J., et al., "Propranolol as an adjunct therapy for hyperthyroid tremor," *Eur Neurol* 1997; 37:182–85.

Hennemann, G., Autonomously Functioning Thyroid Nodules and Other Causes of Thyrotoxicosis. In DeGroot, L., Jameson, J., (Eds) . Endocrinology 5th Ed. Philadelphia: Saunders/Elsevier, 2006, p. 2043–53.

Hoffmann, D., et al., *Medical Herbalism: The Science and Practice of Herbal Medicine.* Rochester, VT: Healing Arts Press, 2003.

Igbal, A., et al., "Hypercalcemia in hyperthyroidism: patterns of serum calcium, parathyroid hormone, and 1,25-dihydroxyvitamin D3 levels during management of thyrotoxicosis," *Endo Crin Pract* 2003; 9:517–21.

Ingbar, S., Possible role for bacterial antigens in the pathogenesis of autoimmune thyroid disease. In Pincheta, A., et al., (Ed.) Thyroid Immunity. New York: Plenum, 1987 p. 35–44.

Joasoo, A., et al., "Viral antibodies and thyrotoxicosis," (letter) . *Lancet* 1975; 2:125.

Kahaly, G., et al., "Cardiac risks of hyperthyroidism in the elderly," *Thyroid* 1998; 8:1165–69.

Kahaly, G. "Stress echocardiography in hyperthyroidism," *Jour Clin Endocrinol Metabol* 1999; 84:2308–13.

Kahaly, G., et al., "Thyroid hormone action in the heart," *Endocr Rev* 2005; 26:704–28.

Kasemsuwan, L., et al. "Recurrent laryngeal nerve paralysis: A complication of thyroidectomy," *Jour Otolaryngol* 1997; 26:365–67.

Kelly, G., "Peripheral metabolism of the thyroid hormones: a review," *Alt Med Rev* 2005; 5(4):307–33.

Kidd, G., et al., "The hypothalamic-pituitary-testicular axis in thyrotoxicosis," *Jour Clin Endocrinol Metabol* 1979; 48:798–802.

Kodall, V., et al,, "Thyrotoxic periodic paralysis: a case report and review of the literature," *Jour Emerg Med* 1999; 17:43–5.

Krassas, G., et al., "A prospective controlled study of the impact of hyperthyroidism on reproductive function in males," *Jour Clin Endocrinol Metab* 2002; 87(8):36667–71.

Krassas, G., et al., "Menstrual disturbances in thyrotoxicosis," Clin Endocrin (Orf) 1994; 40(5):641-44.

Krassas, G., et al., "Thyroid function and human reproductive health," *Endocr Rev* 2010; 31(5):702–55.

Kubota, S., et al., "Serial changes in liver function tests in patients with thyrotoxicosis induced by Grave's disease and painless thyroiditis," *Thyroid* 2008; 18(3):283–87.

Kurnik, D., et al., "Complex drug-drug-disease interactions between amiodarone, warfarin, and the thyroid gland," *Medicine (Baltimore)* 2004; 83:107–13.

Larson, P., et al., The thyroid gland. In Wilson, J., Foster, D., (Eds.) William's Textbook of Endocrinology. 8th Ed. Philadelphia: WB Saunders, 1992, p. 367–487.

Laurberg, P., et al., "Inhibitory effect of various radiographic contrast agents on secretion of thyroxine by the dog thyroid and on peripheral thyroidal deiodination of thyroxine to triiodothyronine," *Jour Endocrinol* 1987; 112:387–90.

Lazarus, J., "Guidelines for the use of radioiodine in the management of hyperthyroidism: A summary. Prepared by the Radioiodine Audit Subcommittee of the Royal College of Physicians Committee on Diabetes and Endocrinology, and the Research Unit of the Royal College of Physicians. JR Coll Physicians Lond 1995; 29:464–69.

Leznoff, A., et al., "Syndrome of idiopathic chronic urticaria and angioedema with thyroid autoimmunity: A study of 90 patients," *Jour Allergy Clin Immunol* 1989; 84:66071.

Liaw, Y., et al., "Hepatic injury during propylthiouracil therapy in patients with hyperthyroidism: A cohort study," *Ann Inter Med* 1993; 118:424–28.

Low-Dog, T., Integrative approach to endocrinology. In Kligler, B., Lee, R., (Eds.) Integrative Medicine: Principles for Practice. New York: McGraw-Hill, 2004, p. 433–55.

Mandel, S., et al., Thyrotoxicosis. In Melmed, S., et al. (Eds.) Williams Textbook of Endocrinology 12th Ed. Philadelphia: Saunders/Elsevier, 2011, p. 362–405.

Marigold, J., et al., "Lugol's iodine: Its effect on thyroid blood flow in patients with thyrotoxicosis," *Brit Jour Surg* 1985; 72:45–7.

Martino, E., et al., "The effects of amiodarone on the thyroid," *Endocr Rev* 2001; 22:240–54.

Max, M., et al., "Early and late complications after thyroid operations," *South Med Jour* 1983; 76:977–80.

"Meikle, A., "The interrelationships between thyroid dysfunction and hypogonadism in men and boys," *Thyroid* 2004; (Suppl 1):517–25.

Menke, T., et al., "Plasma levels of coenzyme Q-10 in children with hyperthyroidism," *Horm Res* 2004; 61:153–58.

"Menstrual disturbances in thyrotoxicosis," *Clin Endocriol (Oxf)*:1994; 40(5):641–44.

Milila, C., et al., "Pulmonary complications of endocrine and metabolic disorders," *Paediatr Respir Rev* 2012; 13(1):23–8.

Miller, M., Disorder of the Thyroid. In Fillit, H., et al., (Eds.) Brocklehurst's Textbook of Geriatric Medicine and Gerontology. 7th Ed. Philadelphia: Saunders/Elsevier, 2010, p. 737–54.

Mohan, H., et al, "Thyroid hormone and parathyroid hormone competing to maintain calcium levels in the presence of vitamin D deficiency," *Thyroid* 2004; 14:789–91.

Mouradian, M., et al., "Diabetes mellitus and thyroid disease," *Diabetes Care* 1983; 6:512–20.

Muldoon, B., et al., "Management of Grave's disease," In Burman, K., and Jonklaas, J., (Eds.) Thyroid Cancer and Other Thyroid Disorders. Endocrinology and Metabolism Clinics of North America, June 2014; 43(2): 495–516.

Mundy, G., et al., "Direct stimulation of bone resorption by thyroid hormones," *Jour Clin Invest* 1976; 58:529–34.

Murray, M., Hyperthyroidism. In Pizzorno, J., Murray, M., (Eds.) Textbook of Natural Medicine. 3rd Ed. St. Louis: Churchhill/Livingstone/Elsevier, 2006, p. 1771–79.

Myers, J., et al., "A correlative study of the cardiac output and the hepatic circulation in hyperthyroidism," *Jour Clin Invest* 1950; 29:1069–77.

Nakazawa, H., et al., "Is there a place for the late cardioversion of atrial fibrillation? A long-term follow-up study of patients with post-thyrotoxic atrial fibrillation," *Eur Heart* Jour 2000; 21:327–33.

Nakazawa, H., et al., "Management of atrial fibrillation in the post-thyrotoxic state," *Amer Jour Med* 1982; 72:903–06.

Napoli, R., "Impact of hyperthyroidism and its correction on vascular reactivity in humans," *Circulation* 2001; 104:3076–80.

Northcote, R., et al., "Continuous 24-hour electrocardiography in thyrotoxicosis before and after treatment," *Amer Heart Jour* 1986; 112:339–44.

Ober, K., "Thyrotoxic periodic paralysis in the United States: report of 7 cases and review of the literature," *Medicine (Baltimore)* 1992; 71:109–120.

Ogura, F., et al., "Serum coenzyme Q-10 levels in thyroid disorders," *Horm Metab Res* 1980; 12:537–40.

Ojamaa, K., et al., "Changes in adenylyl cyclase isoforms as a mechanism for thyroid hormone modulation of cardiac beta-adrenergic receptor responsiveness," *Metabolism* 2000; 49:275–79.

Oliviero, O., et al., "Low selenium status in older adults influences thyroid hormones," *Clin Sci* 1995; 89:637–42.

Panda, S., et al., "Fruit extract of Emblica officinalis ameliorates hyperthyroidism and hepatic lipid peroxidation in mice," *Pharmazie* 2003; 58:753–55.

Pattou, F., et al., "Hypocalcemia following thyroid surgery: Incidence and prediction of outcome," *World Jour Surg* 1998; 22:718–24.

Petersen, P., et al., "Stroke in thyrotoxicosis with atrial fibrillation," *Stoke* 1988; 19:15–18.

Phillips, D., et al., "The geographical distribution of thyrotoxicosis in England according to the presence of absence of TSH-receptor antibodies," *Clin Endocrinol (Oxf)* 1985; 23:283–87.

Pimenta, W., "The assessment of zinc status by the zinc tolerance test and thyroid disease," *Trace Element Med* 1992; 9:34–7.

Pino-Garcia, J., et al., "Regulation of breathing in hyperthyroidism: relationship to hormonal and metabolic changes," *Eur Respir Jour* 1998; 12(2):400–07.

Priest, A., et al., *Herbal Medication.* London: Fowler and Co., 1982.

Sawin, C., et al., "Low serum thyrotoxin concentrations as a risk factor for atrial fibrillation in older persons," *NEJM* 1994; 331:1249–52.

Seven, A., et al., "Lipid peroxidation and vitamin E supplementation in experimental hyperthyroidism," *Clin Chem* 1996; 42:1118–19.

Shenkman, I., et al., "Antibodies to Yersinia enterocolitica in thyroid disease," *Ann Inter Med* 1976; 85:735–39.

Silva, J., "The thermogenic effect of thyroid hormone and its clinical implications," *Amer Intern Med* 2003; 139:205–13.

Solomon, B., et al., "Remission rates with antithyroid drug therapy: Continuing influence of iodine intake?" *Ann Intern Med* 1987; 107:510–12.

Speroff, L., et al., *Clinical Gynecologic Endocrinology and Infertility.* Baltimore: Lippincott, Williams, and Wilkins, 1999.

Stagnaro-Green, A., et al., "Detection of at risk pregnancy by means of highly sensitive assays for thyroid autoantibodies," *JAMA* 1990; 264:1422–25.

Stagnaro-Green, A., et al., "Thyroid autoimmunity and the risk of miscarriage," *Best Pract Res Clin Endocrin Metabol* 2004; 18:167–81.

Tagawa, N., et al., "Serum concentration of androstenediol and androstenediol sulfate in patients with hyperthyroidism and hypothyroidism," *Endocr Jour* 2001; 48:345–54.

Tanlyama, M., et al., "Urinary cortisol metabolites in the assessment of pheripheral thyroid hormone action: application for diagnosis of resistance to thyroid hormone," *Thyroid* 1993; 3:229–33.

Tas, M., et al., "Defects in monocyte polarization and dendritic cell clustering in patients with disease: A putative role for non-specific immunoregulatory factor related to retroviral p15E." *Clin Endocrinol* 1991; 34:441–48.

Tomer, Y., et al., "Infection, thyroid disease and autoimmunity," *Endocr Rev* 1993; 14:107–20.

Tomer, Y., et al., "Thyroglobulin is a thyroid specific gene for the familial autoimmune disease," *Jour Clin Endocrinol Metabol* 2002; 87:404–07.

Trivalle, C., "Differences in the signs and symptoms of hyperthyroidism in older and younger patients," *Jour Amer Geriatr Soc* 1996; 44:50–3.

Valtonen, V., et al., "Serological evidence for the role of bacterial infections in the pathogenesis of thyroid disease," *Acta Med Scand* 1986; 219:105.

Wakasugi, M., et al., "Bone mineral density of patients with hyperthyroidism measured by dual energy X-ray absorption," *Clin Endorinol (Oxf)* 1993; 38:283–86.

Wakasugi, M., et al., "Change in bone mineral density in patients with hyperthyroidism after attainment of euthyroidism by dual energy X-ray absorptiometry," *Thyroid* 1994; 4:179–82.

Weiss, R., et al., *Herbal Medicine,* 2nd Ed. Stuttgart: Thime, 2000.

Wejda, B., et al., "Hip fractures and the thyroid: a case-control study," *Jour Intern Med* 1995; 237:241–47.

Wiersinga, W., et al., "Propranolol and thyroid hormone metabolism," *Thyroid* 1991; 1:273–77.

Winterhoff, H., et al., "Antihormonal effects of plant extract: pharmacodynamic effects of Lithospermum officinale on the thyroid gland of rats; comparison with the effects of iodide," *Horm Met Res* 1983; 15:503–07.

Wober, K., "Iodine and thyroid disease," *Med Clin North Amer* 1991; 75:169–78.

Wood, L., et al., "Autoimmune thyroid disease, left-handedness, and development dyslexia," *Psychoneuroendocrinology* 1992; 17:95–9.

Wu, S., et al., "Changes in circulating iodothyronines in euthyroid and hyperthyroid subjects given ipodate (Oragrafin) an agent for oral cholecystography," *Jour Clin Endocrinol Metabol* 1978; 46:691–97.

Wu, S., et al., "Comparison of sodium ipodate (Oragrafin) and propylthiourcil in early treatment of hyperthyroidism," *Jour Clin Endocrinol Metabol* 1982;54:630–34.

Wu, Z., et al., "The effect of acupuncture on 40 cases of endocrine ophthalmopathy," *Jour Triad Chin Med* 1985; 5:19.

Yu, Wai, Man, C., et al., "Extraocular muscles have fundamentally distinct properties that make them selectively vulnerable to certain disorders," *Neuromuscul Disord* 2005; 15:17–23.

Zaidi, M., et al., "Thyroid-stimulating hormone, thyroid hormones, and bone loss," *Curr Osteoporosis Rep* 2009; 7:47–52.

CHAPTER 4. GRAVES' DISEASE

Alvarado, A., et al., "Lack of association between thyroid function and mitral valve prolapse in Graves' disease," *Braz Jour Med Biol Res* 1990; 23:133–39.

Aufmkok, M., et al., "Extracts and auto-oxidized constituents of certain plants inhibit the receptor-binding and the biological activity of Graves' immunoglobulins," *Endocrinology* 1985; 116:1687–93.

Bennedbaek, F., et al., "The transition of subacute thyroiditis to Graves' disease as evidenced by diagnostic imaging," *Thyroid* 1996; 6:457–59.

Bunevicius, R., et al., "Psychiatric manifestations of Graves' hyperthyroidism: pathophysiology and treatment options," *CNS Drugs* 2006; 20(11):897–909.

Burevicius, R., et al., "Mood and anxiety disorders in women with treated hyperthyroidism and ophthalmopathy caused by Graves' disease," *Gen Hosp Psychiatry* 2005; 27(2):133–9.

Cavan, D., et al., "The HLA association with Graves' disease is sex-specific in Hong Kong Chinese subjects," *Clin Endocrinol (Oxf)* 1994; 40:63–6.

Chang, D., et al., "The effect of preoperative Lugol's iodine on thyroid blood flow in patients with Graves' hyperthyroidism," *Surgery* 1987; 102:1055–61.

Ciampolillo, A., et al., "Retrovirus-like sequences in Graves' disease: Implications for human autoimmunity," *Lancet* 1989; 1:1096–99.

Cooper, D., "Antithyroid drugs for the treatment of hyperthyroidism caused by Graves' disease," *Endocrinol Metab Clin North Amer* 1998; 27:225–47.

Cusick, E., et al., "Outcome of surgery for Graves' disease re-examined," *Brit Jour Surg* 1987; 74:780–83.

Danielsen, E.., et al., "Reduced parietoccipital white matter glutamine measured by proton magnetic resonance spectroscopy in treated Graves' disease patients," *Jour Clin Endocrinol Metab* 2008; 93:3192–98.

Elberling, T., et al., "Reduced myo-inositol and total choline measured with cerebral MRS in acute thyrotoxic Graves' disease," *Neurology* 2003; 60:142–45.

Feldt-Rasmussen, U., et al., "Meta-analysis evaluation of the impact of thyrotropin receptor antibodies on long-term remission after medical therapy of Graves' disease," *Jour Clin Endocrinol Metabol* 1994; 78:98–102.

Fierabravci, A., et al., "Lack of detection of retroviral particles (HIAP-1) in the H9 T cell line co-cultured with thyrocytes of Graves' disease," *Jour Autoimmunity* 2001; 16:457–62.

Hedley, A., et al., "Antithyroid drugs in the treatment of hyperthyroidism of Graves' disease: Long-term follow-u[of 434 patients," Scottish Automated Follow-up Register Group. *Clin Endocrinol (Oxf)* 1989; 31:209018.

Kasuga, Y., et al., "Clinical evaluation of the response to surgical treatment of Graves' disease," *Surg Gynecol Obstet* 1990; 170:327–30.

KItaka, M., et al., "A case with Graves' disease with false hyperthyrotropinemia who developed silent thyroiditis," *Endocrinol Jpn* 1991; 38:667.

Lamberg, R., et al., "Spontaneous hypothyroidism after antithyroid treatment of hyperthyroid Graves' disease," *Jour Endocrinol Invest* 1981; 4:399–402.

Laurberg, P., et al., High incidence of multinodular toxic goitre in the elderly population in a low iodine intake area vs. high incidence of Graves' disease in the young in a high iodine intake area: Comparative surveys of thyrotoxicosis epidemiology in East-Jutland Denmark and Iceland," *Jour Intern Med* 1991; 229:415–20.

Marino, M., et al., Graves' Disease. In DeGroot, L., Jameson, J., (Eds) . Endocrinology 5th Ed. Philadelphia: Saunders/Elsevier, 2006, 1995–28.

Miccoli, P., et al., "Surgical treatment of Graves' disease: Subtotal or total thyroidectomy?" *Surgery* 1996; 120:1020–25.

Muldoon, B., et al., "Management of Grave's disease," In Burman, K., and Jonklaas, J., (Eds.) Thyroid Cancer and Other Thyroid Disorders. Endocrinology and Metabolism Clinics of North America, June 2014; 43(2): 495–516.

Nygaard, B., et al., "Thyrotropin receptor antibodies and Graves' disease, a side-effect of 1–131 treatment in patients with nontoxic goiter," *Jour Clin Endocrinol Metab* 1997; 82:2926–30.

Okamura, K., et al., "Reevaluation of the effects of methylmercaptoimidazole and propylthiouracil in patients with Graves' Disease therapy: European Multicenter Study Group on Antithyroid Drug Treatment," *Jour Clin Endocrinol Metabol* 1993; 76:1516–21.

Pedersen, I., et al., "Serum selenium is low in newly diagnosed Graves' disease: a population-based study," *Clin Endocriol (Oxf)* 2013; 79(4):584–90.

Prummel, M., et al., "The environment and autoimmune thyroid diseases," Eur Jour Endocrinol 2004; 150(5):605-18.

Schleusener, H., et al, "Prospective multicentre study on the prediction of relapse after antithyroid drug treatment in patients with Graves' disease," *Acta Endocrinol (Copenh)* 1989; 120:689–701.

Shen, D., et al., "Long term treatment of Graves' hyperthyroidism," *Jour Clin Endocrinol Metabol* 1985; 61:723–27.

Sonino, N., et al.," Life events in the pathogenesis of Graves' disease. A controlled study," *Acta Endocrinol (Copenh)* 1993; 128:293–96.

Tas, M., et al., "Defects in monocyte polarization and dendritic cell clustering in patients with Graves' disease: A putative role for non-specific immunoregulatory factor related to retroviral p15E." *Clin Endocrinol* 1991; 34:441–48.

Tomer, Y., et al., "Mapping of a major susceptibility locus for Graves' disease (GD-1) to chromosome 14q31," *Jour Clin Endocrinol Metab* 1997; 82:1645–48.

Trzepacz, P., et al., "A psychiatric and neuropsychological study of patients with untreated Graves' disease," *Gen Hosp Psychiatry* 1988; 10:49–55.

Trzepacz, P., et al., "Psychiatric and neuropsychological response to propranolol in Graves' disease," *Biol Psychiatry* 1988; 23:678–88.

van Soestbergen, M., et al., "Recurrence of hyperthyroidism in multinodular goiter after long-term drug therapy: A comparison with Graves' disease," *Jour Endocrinol Invest* 1002; 15:797–800.

Vitti, P., et al., "Clinical features of patients with Graves' disease undergoing remission after antithyroid drug treatment," *Thyroid* 1997; 7:369–75.

Vogel, A., et al., "Affective symptoms and cognitive functions in the acute phase of Graves' thyrotoxicosis," *Psychoneuroendocrinology* 2007; 32(1):36–43.

Vrca, V., et al., "Supplementation with antioxidants in the treatment of Graves' disease: the effect on glutathione peroxidase activity and concentration of selenium," *Clin Chim Acta* 2004; 341:55–63.

Wartofshy, L., "Low remission after therapy for Graves' disease: Possible relation of dietary iodine with antithyroid therapy results," *JAMA* 1973; 226:1083–88.

Yanagawa, T., et al., "CTLA-4 gene polymorphism associated with Graves' disease in a Caucasian population," *Jour Clin Endocrinol Metabol* 1995; 80:41–5.

CHAPTER 5. THYROID DISORDERS CAUSED BY/OR ASSOCIATED WITH HYPERTHYROIDISM AND THYROTOXICOSIS

Aliciguzel, Y., et al., "Erythrocyte, plasma, and serum antioxidant activities in untreated toxic multinodular goiter patients," *Free Rad Biol Med* 2001; 15; 30:665–70.

Bennedbaek, F., et al., "Diagnosis and treatment of the solitary thyroid nodule: Results of a European survey," *Clin Endocrinol (Oxf)* 1999; 50:357–63.

Bennedbaek, F., et al., "Management of the solitary thyroid nodule: Results of a North American survey," *Jour Clin Endocrinol Metab* 2000; 85:2493–98.

Berghout, A., et al., "Comparison of placebo with L-thyroxine alone or with carbimazole for treatment of sporadic non-toxic goitre," *Lancet* 1990; 336:193–97.

Bonnema, S., et al., ""Management of the nontoxic multinodular goiter: A European questionnaire study," *Clin Endocrinol (Oxf)* 2000; 53:5–12.

Bonnema, S., et al., "Management of the nontoxic multinodular goiter: A North American survey," *Jour Clin Endocrinol Metab* 2002; 87:112–17.

Brix, T., et al., "Genetic and environmental factors in the aetilogy of simple goitre," *Ann Med* 2000; 32:153–56.

Burgi, H., et al., "Iodine deficiency diseases in Switzerland one hundred years after Theodor Kocher's survey: A historical review with some new goitre prevalence data," *Acta Endocrinol (Copenh)* 1990; 123:577–90.

Corral, J., et al., "Thyroglobulin gene point mutation associated with non-endemic simple goitre," *Lancet* 1993; 341:462–64.

Dossing, H., et al., "Ultrasound-guided interstitial laser photocoagulation of an autonomous thyroid nodule: The introduction of a novel alternative," *Thyroid* 2003; 13:885.

Elte, J., et al., "The natural history of euthyroid multinodular goitre," *Postgrad Med Jour* 1990; 66:186–190.

Eyre-Brook, I., et al., "The treatment of autonomous functioning thyroid nodules," *Brit Jour Surg* 1982; 69:577.

Hegedis, I., et al., "Management of simple nodular goiter: Current status and future perspectives," *Endocr Rev* 2003; 24:102–32.

Hegedus, L., et al., Multinodular Goiter. In DeGroot, L., Jameson, J., (Eds) . Endocrinology 5th Ed. Philadelphia: Saunders/Elsevier, 2006, p. 2113–27.

Huysmans, D., et al., "Large, compressive goiters treated with radioiodine," *Ann Intern Med* 1994; 121:757–62.

Lippi, F., et al., "Treatment of solitary autonomous thyroid nodules by percutaneous ethanol injection: Results of an Italian multicenter study. The Multicenter Study Group," *Jour Clin Endocrinol Metab* 1996; 81:3261.

Mariotti, S., et al., "Serum thyroid auto-antibodies as a risk factor for development of hypothyroidism after radioactive iodine therapy for single thyroid "hot" nodule," *Acta Endocrinol (Copenh)* 1986; 113:500.

Muldoon, B., et al., "Management of Grave's disease," In Burman, K., and Jonklaas, J., (Eds.) Thyroid Cancer and Other Thyroid Disorders. Endocrinology and Metabolism Clinics of North America, June 2014; 43(2): 495–516.

Nygaard, B., et al., "Radioiodine therapy for multinodular toxic goiter," Arch Intern Med 1999; 159:1364–68.

Nygaard, B., et al., "Transition of nodular toxic goiter to autoimmune hyperthyroidism triggered by I-131 therapy," Thyroid 1999; 9:477–81.

Paracchi, A., et al., "Changes in radioiodine turnover in patients with autonomous thyroid adenoma treated with percutaneous ethanol injection," Jour Nucl Med 1998; 39:1012.

Spiezia, S., et al., "Ultrasound-guided laser thermal ablation in the treatment of autonomous hyperfunctioning thyroid nodules and compressive nontoxic nodular goiter," Thyroid 2003; 13:941.

CHAPTER 6. THYROID HORMONES AND YOUR MEMORY

Alzoubi, K., et al., "Levothyroxine restores hypothyroidism-induced impairment of LTP of hippocampal CA1: electrophysiological and molecular studies," Exp Neurol 2005; 195:330–41.

Bauer, M., et al., "Brain glucose metabolism in hypothyroidism: a positron emission tomography study before and after thyroid hormone replacement therapy," Jour Clin Endocrinol Metab 2009; 94:2922–29.

Bemal, J., "Thyroid hormones and brain development," Vit Horm 2005; 71:95–122.

Burmeister, L., et al., "Hypothyroidism and cognition: preliminary evidence for a specific defect in memory," Thyroid 2001; 11:1177–85.

Correla, N., et al., "Evidence for a specific defect in hippocampal memory in overt and subclinical hypothyroidism," Jour Clin Endocrinol Metab 2009; 94:3789–97.

Desouza, L., et al., "Thyroid hormone regulates hippocampal neurogenesis in the adult rat brain," Mol Cell Neurosci 2005; 29:414–26.

Ehninger, D., et al., "Paradoxical effects of learning the Morris water maze on adult hippocampal neurogenesis in mice may be explained by a combination of stress and physical activity," genes Brain Behav 2006; 5:29–39.

Fernandez-Lamo I., et al., "Effects of thyroid hormone replacement on associative learning and hippocampal synaptic plasticity in adult hypothyroid rats," Eur Jour Neurosci 2009; 30:679–92.

Forti, P., et al., Serum thyroid stimulating hormone as a predictor of cognitive impairment in an elderly cohort," Gerontology 2011; Epub ahead of print, accessed October 9, 2011.

Gerges, N., et al., "Hypothyroidism impairs late LTP in CA1 region but not dentate gyrus of the intact rat hippocampus: MAPK involvement," Hippocampus 2004; 14:40–5.

He, X., et al., "Functional magnetic resource imaging assessment of altered brain function in hypothyroidism during working memory processing," Eur Jour Endocrinol 2011; 164(6):951–59.

Johnson, L., et al., "The influence of thyroid function on cognition in a sample of ethnically diverse, rural-dwelling women: a project FRONTIER study," *Jour Neuropsychiatry Clin Neurosci* 2011; 23(2):219–22.

Koromilas, C., et al., "Structural and functional alterations in the hippocampus due to hypothyroidism," *Metab Brain Dis* 2010; 25:339–54.

Mennemeier, M., et al., "Memory, mood and measurement in hypothyroidism," *Jour Clin Exp Neuropsychol* 1993; 822–31.

Miller, K., et al., "Memory improvement with treatment of hypothyroidism," *Jour Neurosci* 2006; 116:895–906.

Miller, K., et al., "Verbal memory retrieval deficits associated with untreated hypothyroidism," Jour Neuropsychiatry *Clin Neurosci* 2007;19:132–36.

Morreale de Escobar, G., et al., "Is neuropsychological development related to maternal hypothyroidism or to maternal hypothyroxinemia," *Jour Clin Endocriol Metab* 2000; 85:3975–87.

Osterweil, D., et al., "Cognitive function in non-demented older adults with hypothyroidism," *Jour Amer Geriatr Soc* 1992; 40:325–35.

Rivas, M., et al., "Thyroid hormones, learning and memory," *Genes, Brain Behavior* 2007; 6(Suppl 1): 40–44.

Samuels, M., "Cognitive function in untreated hypothyroidism and hyperthyroidism," *Currr Opin Endocrinol Diabetes Obes* 2006; 15:429–33.

Samuels, M., "Thyroid disease and cognition," In Burman, K., and Jonklaas, J., (Eds.) Thyroid Cancer and Other Thyroid Disorders. Endocrinology and Metabolism Clinics of North America, June 2014; 43(2):529–43.

Santisteban, P., et al., "Thyroid development and effect on the nervous system," *Rev Endocr Metab Disord* 2005; 6:217–28.

Shors, T., et al., "Neurogenesis may relate to some but not all types of hippocampal-dependent learning," *Hippocampus* 2002; 12:578–84.

Smith, J., et al., "Thyroid hormones, brain function and cognition: a brief review," *Neurosci Biobehav Rev* 2002; 26:45–60.

Smith, P., *What You Must Know About Memory Loss and How You Can Stop It.* Garden City Park, NY: Square One Publishers, 2014.

Wilcoxon, J., et al., "Behavioral inhibition and impaired spatial learning and memory in hypothyroid mice lacking thyroid hormone receptor alpha," *Behav Brain Res* 2007; 177(1):109–16.

Zhu, D., et al., "fMRI revealed neural substrate for reversible working memory dysfunction in subclinical hypothyroidism," *Brain* 2006; 129:2923–30.

CHAPTER 7. THYROID DYSFUNCTION AND YOUR MOOD

Burevicius, R., et al., "Mood and anxiety disorders in women with treated hyperthyroidism and ophthalmopathy caused by Graves' disease," *Gen Hosp Psychiatry* 2005; 27(2):133–9.

Carta, M., et al., "The link between thyroid autoimmunity (antithyroid peroxidase autoantibodies) with anxiety and mood disorders in the community: a field of interest in public health in the future," *BMC Psychiatry* 2004; 4:25.

Constant, E., et al., "Anxiety and depression, attention and executive functions in hypothyroidism," *Jour Int Neuropsychol Soc* 2005; 11:535–44.

Egede, I., et al., "Depression and all-cause and coronary heart disease mortality among adults with and without diabetes," *Diabetes Care* 2005; 28:1339–45.

Esposito, S., et al.,, "The thyroid axis and mood disorders: overview and future prospects," *Psychopharmacol Bull* 1997; 33:205–17.

Frasure-Smith, M., et al., "Recent evidence linking coronary heart disease and depression," *Can Jour Psychiatry* 2006; 51:730–37.

Lecrubier, Y., "Widespread underrecognition and treatment of anxiety and mood disorders: results from 3 European studies," *Jour Clin Psychiatry* 2007; 68(Suppl 2):36–41.

Mennemeier, M., et al., "Memory, mood and measurement in hypothyroidism," *Jour Clin Exp Neuropsychol* 1993; 822–31.

Montero-Pedrazuela, A., et al., "Modulation of adult hippocampal neurogenesis by thyroid hormones: implications in depressive-like behavior," *Mol Psychiatry* 2006; 11:361–71.

Rugulies, R., "Depression as a predictor for coronary heart disease: a review and meta-analysis," *Amer Jour Prev Med* 2002; 23:51–61.

Samuels, M., et al., "Health status, mood, and cognition in experimentally induced subclinical hypothyroidism," *Jour Clin Endocrinol Metab* 2007; 92:2545–51.

Schreckenberger, M.,, et al., "Positron emission tomography reveals correlations between brain metabolism and mood changes in hyperthyroidism," *Jour Clin Endocrinol Metab* 2006; 91:4786–91.

Van Boxtel, M., et al., "Thyroid function, depressed mood, and cognitive performance in older individuals: The Maastricht Aging Study," *Psychoneuroendocrinology* 2004; 29:891–98.

CHAPTER 8. THYROID HORMONES AND YOUR HEART

Althaus, U., et al., "LDL/HDL-changes in subclinical hypothyroidism: possible risk factors for coronary heart disease," *Clin Endocrinol* 1989; 28:157–63.

Alvarado, A., et al., "Lack of association between thyroid function and mitral valve prolapse in Graves' disease," *Braz Jour Med Biol Res* 1990; 23:133–39.

Asvold, B., et al., "Thyrotropin levels and risk of fatal coronary heart disease: the HUNT study," Arch Intern Med 2008; 168:855–60.

Biondi, B., et al., Effects of subclinical thyroid dysfunction on the heart," *Ann Internal* 2002; 137:904–14.

Brauman, A., et al., "Prevalence of mitral valve prolapse in chronic lymphocytic thyroiditis and nongoitrous hypothyroidism," *Cardiology* 1988; 75:269–73.

Burggraaf J., et al., "Sympathovagal imbalance in hyperthyroidism" *Amer Jour Physiol Endocrinol Metabol* 2001; 281:E190–95.

Cappola, A., et al., "Thyroid status, cardiovascular risk, and mortality in older adults," *JAMA* 2006; 295:1033–41.

Chen, L., et al., "Depressed mitochondrial fusion in heart failure," *Circulation* 2007; 116:259.

Coceani, M., et al., "Thyroid hormone and coronary artery disease: from clinical correlations to prognostic implications," *Clin Cardiol* 2009; 32:389–85.

Corral-Debrinski, M., et al., "Association of mitochondrial DNA damage with aging and coronary atherosclerotic heart disease," *Mutat Res* 1992; 275(3–6):169–80.

Dahi, P., "Thyrotoxic cardiac disease," *Curr Heart Fail Rep* 2008; 5:170–76.

Danzi, S., et al., "Alterations in thyroid hormones with accompany cardiovascular diseases," *Clinical Thyroidology* 2009; 21:3–5.

Danzi, S., et al., "Thyroid hormone and blood pressure regulation," *Curr Hypertens Rep* 2003; 5:513–20.

Danzi, S., et al., "Thyroid hormone and the cardiovascular system," *Med Clin North Amer* 2012; 96:257–68.

Danzi, S., et al., "Triiodothyronine mediated myosin heavy chain gene transcription in the heart," *Amer Jour Physiol Heart Circ Physiol* 2003; 284:H2263.

Danzi, S., et al., "Changes in thyroid hormone metabolism and gene expression in the failing heart: therapeutic implications." In Iervasi, G., Pingitore, A., (Eds.) Thyroid and Heart Failure: From Pathophysiology to Clinics. Italy: Springer-Verlag, 2009, p. 97–107.

DeGroot, L., "Non-thyroid illness syndrome is a manifestation of hypothalamic-pituitary dysfunction, and in view of current evidence, should be treated with appropriate replacement therapies," *Crit Care Clin* 2006; 22:57–86.

Deyssig, R., et al., "Ingestion of androgenic-anabolic steroids induces mild thyroidal impairment in male body builders," *Jour Clin Endocrinol Metab* 1993; 76(4):1069–71.

Dillmann, W., "Cellular action of thyroid hormone on the heart," *Thyroid* 2012; 12:447–52.

Egede, I., et al., "Depression and all-cause and coronary heart disease mortality among adults with and without diabetes," *Diabetes Care* 2005; 28:1339–45.

Fazio, S., et al., "Effects of thyroid hormone on the cardiovascular system," *Recent Prog Horm Res* 2004; 59:31–50.

Frasure-Smith, M., et al., "Recent evidence linking coronary heart disease and depression," *Can Jour Psychiatry* 2006; 51:730–37.

Friberg, L., et al., "Association between increased levels of reverse triiodothyronine and mortality after acute myocardial infarction," *Amer Jour Med* 2001; 111(9):699–703.

Gerdes, A., et al., "Thyroid replacement therapy and heart failure," *Circulation* 2010; 122:385–93.

Hak, A., et al., "Subclinical hypothyroidism is an independent risk factor for atherosclerosis and myocardial infarction in elderly women: The Rotterdam Study," *Ann Int Med* 2000; 132 (4):270–78.

Hamilton, M., et al., "Altered thyroid hormone metabolism in advance heart failure," *Jour Amer Coll Cardiol* 1990; 16:91–5.

Hamilton, M., et al., "Safety and hemodynamic effects of IV triiodothyronine in advanced congestive heart failure," *Amer Jour Card* 1998; 81(4):443–47.

Hamilton, M., et al., "Thyroid hormonal abnormalities in heart failure: possibilities for therapy," *Thyroid* 1996; 6(5):527–29.

Henderson, K., et al., "Physiological replacement of T3 improves left ventricular function in an animal model of myocardial infarction-induced congestive heart failure," *Circ Heart Fail* 2009; 2:243–52.

Iacoviello, M., et al., "Prognostic role of sub-clinical hypothyroidism in chronic heart failure outpatients," *Curr Pharm Des* 2008; 14:2686–92.

Imaizumi, M., et al., "Risk for ischemic heart disease and all-cause mortality in subclinical hypothyroidism," *Jour Clin Endocrinol Metab* 2004; 89:3365–70.

Ismail, H., "Reversible pulmonary hypertension and isolated right-sided heart failure associated with hyperthyroidism," *Jour Gen Intern Med* 2007; 22:148–50.

Kahaly, G. "Stress echocardiography in hyperthyroidism," *Jour Clin Endocrinol Metabol* 1999; 84:2308–13.

Kahaly, G., et al., "Cardiac risks of hyperthyroidism in the elderly," *Thyroid* 1998; 8:1165–69.

Kahaly, G., et al., "Thyroid hormone action in the heart," *Endocr Rev* 2005; 26:704–28.

Klein, I., "Endocrine disorders and cardiovascular disease," In: Bonow, R., et al (Eds.) Braunwald's Heart Disease. 9th Ed. St. Louis: WB Saunders and Company, 2011, p. 1829–43.

Klein, I., et al., "Thyroid disease and the heart," *Circulation* 2007; 116:1725–35.

Klein, I., et al., "Thyroid hormone and the cardiovascular system," *NEJM* 2001; 344:501–09.

Klein, I., et al., The cardiovascular system in thyrotoxicosis. In Braverman, L., and Utiger, R., (Eds) . Werner & Ingbar's The Thyroid: A Fundamental and Clinical Text. 10th Ed. Philadelphia: Lippincott Williams & Wilkins, 2012, p. 559–68.

Kvetny, J., et al., "Subclinical hypothyroidism is associated with a low-grade inflammation, increased triglyceride levels and predicts cardiovascular disease in males below 50 years," *Clin Endocrinol (Oxf)* 2004; 61:232–38.

Lambrinoudaki, I., et al., "High normal thyroid-stimulating hormone is associated with arterial stiffness in healthy postmenopausal women," *Jour Hypertension* 2012; 30(3):592–99.

Lervasi, G., et al., "Association between increased mortality and mild thyroid dysfunction in cardiac patients," *Arch Intern Med* 2007; 167:1526–32.

Lervasi, G., et al., "Low-T3 syndrome: a strong prognostic predictor of death in patients with heart disease," *Circulation* 2003; 107:708–13.

Lubrano, V., et al., "Relationship between triiodothyronine and proinflammatory cytokines in chronic heart failure," *Biomed Pharmacother* 2010; 64:165–69.

Nakazawa, H., et al., "Is there a place for the late cardioversion of atrial fibrillation? A long-term follow-up study of patients with post-thyrotoxic atrial fibrillation," *Eur Heart Jour* 2000; 21:327–33.

Nakazawa, H., et al., "Management of atrial fibrillation in the post-thyrotoxic state," *Amer Jour Med* 1982; 72:903–06.

Napoli, R., "Impact of hyperthyroidism and its correction on vascular reactivity in humans," *Circulation* 2001; 104:3076–80.

Newman, C., et al., "Amiodarone and the thyroid: A practical guide to the management of thyroid dysfunction induced by amiodarone therapy," *Heart* 1998; 79:121–27.

Nicolini, G., et al., "New insights into mechanisms of cardioprotection mediated by thyroid hormones," *Jour Thyroid Res* 2013; 264387.

Northcote, R., et al., "Continuous 24-hour electrocardiography in thyrotoxicosis before and after treatment," *Amer Heart Jour* 1986; 112:339–44.

Parle, J., et al., "Prediction of all-cause and cardiovascular mortality in elderly people from one low serum thyrotropin result: a 10-year cohort study," *Lancet* 2001; 358:861.

Petersen, P., et al., "Stroke in thyrotoxicosis with atrial fibrillation," *Stroke* 1988; 19:15–18.

Pingitore, A., et al., "Acute effects of triiodothyronine (T3) replacement therapy in patients with chronic heart failure and low-T3 syndrome: a randomized, placebo-controlled study," *Jour Clin Endocrinol Metab* 2008; 93:1351–58.

Poi, C., et al.,, "Cardiomyocyte-specific inactivation of thyroid hormone in pathologic ventricular hypertrophy: an adaptive response or part of the problem?" *Heart Fail Rev* 2010; 15:133–42.

Portman, M., "Thyroid hormone regulation of heart metabolism," *Thyroid* 2008; 18:217–25.

Razvi, S., et al., "Levothyroxine treatment of subclinical hypothyroidism, fatal and nonfatal cardiovascular events, and mortality," *Arch Intern Med* 2012; 172:811–17.

Razvi, S., et al., "The beneficial effect of L-thyroxine on cardiovascular risk factors, endothelial function and quality of life in subclinical hypothyroidism: randomized crossover trial," *Jour Clin Endocrinol Metab* 2007; 92:1715–23.

Rodondi, N., et al., "Subclinical hypothyroidism and the risk of coronary heart disease and mortality," *JAMA* 2010; 304:1365.

Roef, G., et al., "Thyroid hormone levels within the reference range are associated with heart rate, cardiac structure, and function in middle-aged men and women," *Thyroid* 2013; 23:947–54.

Rugulies, R., "Depression as a predictor for coronary heart disease: a review and meta-analysis," *Amer Jour Prev Med* 2002; 23:51–61.

Sawin, C., et al., "Low serum thyrotoxin concentrations as a risk factor for atrial fibrillation in older persons," *NEJM* 1994; 331:1249–52.

Shimoyama, N., et al., "Serum thyroid hormone levels correlate with cardiac function and ventricular tachyarrhythmia in patients with chronic heart failure," *Jour Card* 1993; 23(2):205–13.

Zhang, B., et al., "A low free T3 level as a prognostic marker in patients with acute myocardial infarctions," *Intern Med* 2012; 51:3009–15.

CHAPTER 9. THYROID HORMONES AND DIGESTIVE HEALTH

Berkson, D., *Healthy Digestion the Natural Way.* New York: John Wiley & Sons, 2000.

Graham, D., et al., "Why do apparently healthy people use antacid tablets?" *Amer Jour Gastroenterol* 1983; 78(5):257–60.

Gurlek, A., et al., "Liver tests in hyperthyroidism: effect of antithyroid therapy," *Jour Clin Gastroenterol* 1997; 24:180–83.

Kubota, S., et al., "Serial changes in liver function tests in patients with thyrotoxicosis induced by Grave's disease and painless thyroiditis," *Thyroid* 2008; 18(3):283–87.

Rao, R., et al, "Recent advances in alcoholic liver disease: Role of intestinal permeability and endotoxemia in alcoholic liver disease," *Amer Jour of Physiology, Gastrointestinal and Liver Physiology* 2004; 286(6):G881-G884.

CHAPTER 10. THE THYROID AND CANCER

American Cancer Society. Cancer Facts & Figures 2014. Atlanta: American Cancer Society; 2014.

American Cancer Society: Cancer Facts and Figures, 2015. Atlanta, GA, America Cancer Society; 2015

Brown, A., et al., "Radioactive treatment of metastatic thyroid carcinoma: The Royal Marsden Hospital Experience," *Brit Jour Radiol* 1984; 57:323.

Cardis, E., et al., "Risk of thyroid cancer after exposure to 131 I in childhood," *Jour Natl Cancer Inst* 2005; 97(10):724–32.

Carling, T., et al., Thyroid Tumors. In Devita, V., Lawrence, T., Rosenberg, S., (Eds.) Cancer: Principles and Practice of Oncology. 9th Ed. Philadelphia: Lippincott Williams & Wilkins, 2011.

Danzi, S., et al., Thyroid Disease and the Cardiovascular System. In Burman, K., and Jonklaas, J., (Eds.) Thyroid Cancer and Other Thyroid Disorders. Endocrinology and Metabolism Clinics of North America, June 2014; 43(2):517–28.

Halman, K., "Influence of age and sex on incidence and prognosis of thyroid cancer: 344 cases followed for ten years," *Cancer* 1966; 19:1534–41.

Harach, H., et al., "Thyroid cancer and thyroiditis in the goitrous region of Salta, Argentina, before and after iodine prophylaxis," *Clin Endocrin* 1995; 43:701–06.

Hay, I., "Papillary thyroid carcinoma," *Endocrinol Metab Clin North Amer* 1990; 19:545.

Holden, R., et al., "An immunological model connecting the pathogenesis of stress, depression, and carcinoma," *Med Hypotheses* 1998; 51:309–14.

Hundahl, S., et al., "A National Cancer Base report on 53,856 cases of thyroid carcinoma treated in the US, 1985–1995," *Cancer* 83(12):2638–48.

Iribarren, C., et al., "Cohort study of thyroid cancer in a San Francisco Bay area population," *Int Jour Cancer* 2001; 93(5):745–50.

Kang, K., et al., "Prevalence and rusk of cancer of focal thyroid incidentaloma identified by 18F-fluorodeoxyglucose positron emission tomography for metastasis evaluation and cancer screening in healthy subjects," *Jour Clin Endocrinol Metab* 2003; 88:4100–04.

Khoo, M., et al., "Thyroid calcification and its association with thyroid carcinoma," *Head Neck* 2002; 24(7):651–55.

Massin, J., et al., "Pulmonary metastases in differentiated thyroid carcinoma: Study of 58 cases with implications for the primary treatment," 1984; 53:982–87.

Maxon, H., et al., "Radioiodine-131 in the diagnosis and treatment of metastatic well differentiated thyroid cancer," *Endocrinol Metab Clin North Amer* 1990; 19:685–718.

Mazzaferri, E., "Impact of initial tumor features and treatment selected on the long-term course of differentiated thyroid cancer," *Thyroid Today* 1995; 18(3):1.

Mazzaferri, E., et al., "Papillary thyroid carcinoma: A 10-year follow-up report of the impact of therapy in 576 patients," *Amer Jour Med* 1981; 70:511–18.

Mazzaferri, E., et al., "Papillary thyroid carcinoma: The impact of therapy in 576 patients," *Medicine (Baltimore)* , 1977, 56:171–96.

Nagataki, S., and Torizuka, K., (Eds.) The Thyroid. New York: Elsevier, 1988, p. 685.

Paul, S., et al., "Thyrotoxicosis caused by thyroid cancer," *Endocrinol Metab Clin North Amer* 1990; 19:593.

Nakashima, T., et al., "Predominant T3 synthesis in the metastatic thyroid carcinoma in a patient with T3-toxicosis," *Metabolism* 1981; 30:327.

Niederle, B., et al., "Surgical treatment of distant metastases in differentiated thyroic cancer: Indication and results," *Surgery* 1986; 100:1088.

Pacini, F., et al., "Diagnostic value of a single serum tg determination on and off thyroid suppressive therapy in the follow-up of differentiated thyroid cancer," *Clin Endocrinol (Oxf)* 1985; 23:405.

Pacini, F., et al., "Prevalence of thyroid autoantibodies in children and adolescents from Belarus exposed to the Chernobyl radioactive fallout," *Lancet* 1998; 352(9130):763–66.

Pacini, F., et al., "Serum Thyroglobulin Determination in Thyroid Cancer: A Ten Years Experience. In Nagataki, S., and Torizuka, K., (Eds.) The Thyroid. New York: Elsevier, 1988; p. 685.

Ronson, A., "Stress and allostatic load: perspectives in psycho-oncology," *Bull Cancer* 2006; 93:289–95.

Samaan, N., et al., "Impact of therapy for differentiated carcinoma of the thyroid: An analysis of 706 cases," *Jour Clin Endocrinol Metab* 1983; 56:1131–38.

Samaan, N., et al., "Pulmonary metastasis of differentiated thyroid carcinoma: Treatment results in 101 patients," *Jour Clin Endocrinol Metab* 1985; 60:376.

Schlumberger, M., et al., "Long-term results of treatment of 238 patients with lung and bone metastases from differentiated thyroid carcinoma," *Jour Clin Endocrinol Metab* 1986; 63:960.

Schlumberger, M., et al., 131-1 and External Radiation in the Treatment of Local and Metastatic Thyroid Cancer. In Falk, S., (Ed.) Thyroid Disease. New York: Raven 1990, p. 537.

Simpson, W., et al., "Papillary and follicular thyroid cancer: Prognostic factors in 1578 patients," *Amer Jour Med* 1987; 83:479.

Sosa JA, Hanna J, Lanman RB, Robinson KA, Ladenson PW. Increases in thyroid nodule fine needle aspirations, surgeries and diagnoses of thyroid cancer in the United States. American Association of Endocrine Surgeons 34th Annual Meeting, Apr 14–16, 2013. Chicago, Ill. (oral abstract) .

Tennvall, J., et al., "Is the EORTC prognostic index of thyroid cancer valid in differentiated thyroid cancer? Retrospective multivariate analysis of differentiated thyroid carcinoma with long follow-up," *Cancer* 1986; 57(7):1405–14.

Tollin, S., et al., "The use of fine-needle aspiration biopsy under ultrasound guidance to assess the risk of malignancy in patients with a multinodular goiter," *Thyroid* 2000; 10:235–41.

Tronko, M., et al.,, "A cohort study of thyroid cancer and other thyroid diseases after the Chornobyl accident: thyroid cancer in Ukraine detected during first screening," *Jour Natl Cancer Inst* 2006; 98(13):894–903.

Wallace, D., "A mitochondrial paradigm of metabolic and degenerative diseases, aging and cancer: a dawn for evolutionary medicine," *Ann Rev Genetics* 2005; 39(1):359–407.

About the Author

Pamela Wartian Smith, M.D., MPH, MS spent her first twenty years of practice as an emergency room physician with the Detroit Medical Center and then the next sixteen years as an Anti-Aging/Metabolic Medicine specialist. She is a diplomat of the Board of the American Academy of Anti-Aging Physicians and is an internationally known speaker and author on the subject of Personalized Medicine. She also holds a Master's in Public Health Degree along with a Master's Degree in Metabolic and Nutritional Medicine.

Dr. Smith has been featured on CNN, PBS, and many other television networks, has been interviewed in numerous consumer magazines, and has hosted two of her own radio shows. She is a regular contributor for Fox News Radio. She is currently the Director of the Center for Personalized Medicine and the founder and Director of The Fellowship in Anti-Aging, Regenerative, and Functional Medicine. Dr. Smith is also the co-director of the Master's Program in Metabolic and Nutritional Medicine at the Morsani College of Medicine at the University of South Florida.

Dr. Smith is the author of the best-selling books *What You Must Know About Vitamins, Minerals, Herbs & More*, *What You Must Know about Women's Hormones*, *Why You Can't Lose Weight.*, and *What You Must Know About Memory Loss and How You Can Stop It.*

Index

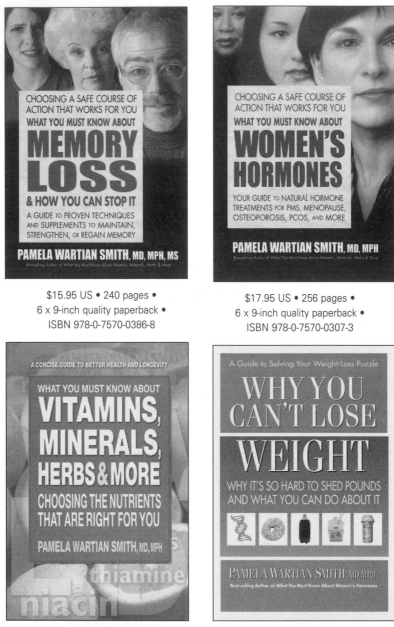